Burning Up, Frozen Out

What Every Man Needs to Know About the Menopause (But No One Told You)

JOE WARNER AND ROB KEMP

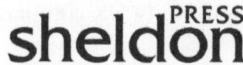

First published in Great Britain by Sheldon Press in 2026
An imprint of John Murray Press

1

Copyright © Joe Warner and Rob Kemp 2026

The right of Joe Warner and Rob Kemp to be identified as the Authors of the Work has been asserted by them in accordance with the Copyright, Designs and Patents Act 1988.

Illustrations © Andrew Sumner

The acknowledgements constitute an extension of this copyright page.

All rights reserved. No part of this publication may be reproduced, stored in a retrieval system, or transmitted, in any form or by any means without the prior written permission of the publisher, nor be otherwise circulated in any form of binding or cover other than that in which it is published and without a similar condition being imposed on the subsequent purchaser.

This book is for information or educational purposes only and is not intended to act as a substitute for medical advice or treatment. Any person with a condition requiring medical attention should consult a qualified medical practitioner or suitable therapist.

A CIP catalogue record for this title is available from the British Library

Trade Paperback ISBN 978 1 399 82665 5
ebook ISBN 978 1 399 82666 2

Typeset by KnowledgeWorks Global Ltd.

Printed and bound in Great Britain by Clays Ltd, Elcograf S.p.A.

John Murray Press policy is to use papers that are natural, renewable and recyclable products and made from wood grown in sustainable forests. The logging and manufacturing processes are expected to conform to the environmental regulations of the country of origin.

John Murray Press	Sheldon Press
Carmelite House	Hachette Book Group
50 Victoria Embankment	123 South Broad Street
London EC4Y 0DZ	Ste 2750
	Philadelphia, PA 19109, USA

www.sheldonpress.co.uk

John Murray Press, part of Hodder & Stoughton Limited
An Hachette UK company

The authorised representative in the EEA is Hachette Ireland, 8 Castlecourt Centre, Dublin 15, D15 XTP3, Ireland (email: info@hbgi.ie)

Praise for *Burning Up, Frozen Out*

'An invaluable manual; no married man should even think of approaching middle age without it.'

Giles Coren, broadcaster and *Times* columnist

'*Burning Up, Frozen Out* is a must-read for any man who wants to truly understand and support the women in his life through menopause. Joe Warner and Rob Kemp break down the science, emotions, and realities with clarity and compassion. This book opens the door to better conversations, deeper empathy, and shared understanding; a vital step toward changing how we all think and talk about menopause.'

Dr Mary Claire Haver, MD, author of *The New Menopause*

'Every man should read and learn – this book has been so well-written and impressively researched!'

Dr Louise Newson, GP and leading menopause specialist

'This is the midlife Bible for both men and women. It's the book I wish my partner had had when I was struggling with menopause symptoms. Clear, funny and potentially a lifesaver, everyone should read it.'

Fiona Clark, author of *Menowars* and founder of the Menopause Research & Education Fund

'Essential reading for every man who cares about a woman.'

Ian Marber, nutrition therapist, consultant and best-selling author

'Men – ignore this book at your peril. Whether you're neck-deep in menopause madness or bracing for the storm ahead, this is your survival manual: entertaining, informative and laugh-out-loud funny. It could be the one thing that saves your sanity – and your relationship.'

Jon Lipsey, former editor-in-chief, *Men's Fitness*

'As a Registered Nutritionist, I see in my clinic how vital it is for couples to navigate midlife and menopause with understanding, compassion and evidence-based guidance. Joe and Rob have created a clear, practical and relatable guide that not only helps men understand the menopause, but also strengthens relationships at a stage of life when connection matters most. *Burning Up, Frozen Out* will make a real difference for so many couples.'

Rhiannon Lambert, registered nutritionist, *Sunday Times* best-selling author and founder of Rhitrition

'Puts the men into menopause and explains with science what's happening to your loved one.'

Phil Williams, broadcaster and BBC Radio 2 Presenter

'Joe and Rob have written an essential and entertaining book that filled holes in my knowledge I didn't know existed. They approach the topic with a great deal of compassion and a thirst for knowledge that's infectious, and it's funny too! Everyone should read it.'

Nick-Harris Fry, health and fitness journalist, *Tom's Guide*

'As a woman soon approaching perimenopause, I want both me and my husband to be prepared as possible for whatever tumult lies ahead. Ignoring something doesn't make it go away, and I'm so glad to see it being openly discussed with the compassion and nuance the topic deserves.'

Liv Boeree, science broadcaster, writer, TED speaker and World Series of Poker champion

'THIS IS SO IMPORTANT. Thank you to Joe Warner for providing us with the tools to stay connected through the challenges of menopause and for recognizing that while this life change happens in women's bodies, its impact on our relationships is profound. Joe's advocacy for communication and understanding in this book will save relationships.'

Christine D'Ercole, Peloton instructor and masters world champion cyclist

'This is the essential guide for any man wishing to understand menopause better, told from a man's perspective. It will also give you a fundamental insight into your own hormones and helps us appreciate that we are not that different after all.'

Dr Jeff Foster, GP and men's health specialist

'This is the book that every partner needs to read. Navigating menopause can be lonely for everyone, especially when you don't know what they are going through or how to support them. Joe has put the guide you need in the pages of this book. A must-read.'

Kate Rowe-Ham, menopause coach and founder of Owning Your Menopause

'Menopause impacts everyone, yet men are so often left out of the conversation. This book finally gives them the tools and confidence to navigate this chapter side-by-side with their partners.'

Jessica Barac, menopause advocate and founder of What The Menopause

'Yes! A book that lifts the lid on the menopause conversation and brings men into the story with honesty, humour and hope. It smashes the silence around menopause and hands men the clarity and confidence to show up as true partners. It's practical, powerful and essential.'

Jaz-Ampaw Farr, award-winning speaker, author and educator

'This book is a real game-changer – clear, compassionate, and brilliantly practical. Joe and Rob strip away the confusion and give couples the tools to face menopause together with confidence, understanding, and real connection. Every man who reads it will feel better equipped to support the woman he loves, and every woman will feel the difference.'

Nigel Denby, registered dietitian, author, broadcaster, and co-founder of Harley Street at Home Menopause

'If your partner has no idea what's happening to you, why you cried when you couldn't find your car keys and then shouted at the cat, buy them this book. Immediately.'

Cheryl Hersey, director, Action PR fitness and wellness group

'Essential reading for any man who wants to understand menopause and support his partner through it. Practical, honest and emotionally intelligent, this book shows how navigating this life stage together can deepen connection, strengthen empathy and enhance your relationship rather than pull you apart.'

Dr Benjamin Davis, GP and men's health specialist

'This book is a treasure-trove of information, written in an engaging manner, with insights relatable to men seeking to understand the menopause. Whether you are a husband, son, friend or colleague, this book will help you be menopause-aware.'

Dr Nicky Keay, hormone health expert and honorary clinical lecturer at UCL

'This book is a must-read for any man who is struggling to understand the menopause and the impact can have on their relationships.'

Lucy Cavendish, relationships counsellor,
author of *How to have Extraordinary Relationships*

*For Lucy and Jack – to the moon and back.
For my mum Chrissy and my niece Lyra –
may tomorrow be brighter than today.
Joe*

*This book is dedicated to the hot, the bothered,
the sleepless, and the brave – this one's for you
(and for the people who live with you).
Rob*

Contents

About the authors ix

Introduction xi

Part 1: Knowledge

1 Your time to shine: How to be the everyday hero she needs 3
2 What the hell is happening? Welcome to the hormone horror show 11
3 Is it getting hot in here? Spotting the signs before she does 29
4 OK, but what about me? Men, mojo and the midlife crisis 45

Part 2: Communication

5 Riding the emotional rollercoaster: Keeping your cool when everything's up in the air 69
6 Breaking the ice: How to talk without making things worse 79
7 Dealing with the doctor: Making sure she's taken seriously 95
8 Walking the treatment tightrope: Getting her the support she needs faster 115

Part 3: Power

9 Stress less and sleep deep: Rapidly recharge both body and mind 141
10 Eat smarter: Good mood food for hormones, health and happiness 171
11 Move more: Exercise for strength, sanity and self-esteem 193
12 Rekindle romance: Getting your love life back on track 221

Afterword 235

References 237

Acknowledgements 291

Index 297

About the authors

Joe Warner is an award-winning journalist and best-selling author. The former editorial director of *Men's Fitness* magazine, he has spent more than two decades working across print, digital and broadcast media, writing extensively about men's and women's health, fitness and wellbeing. He's a regular guest expert on national and international TV, radio, podcasts and in the press. Drop him a line at burningupfrozenout.com or on Instagram (@JoeWarnerUK).

Rob Kemp is a freelance journalist and author of seven non-fiction books, including the Amazon best-selling *The Expectant Dad's Survival Guide*, *The New Dad's Survival Guide* and *The Good Guys: 50 Heroes Who Changed the World with Kindness*. He has written extensively about men's health, parenting and sport for more than 30 years. Get in touch with him at robkempauthor.com or Instagram (@RobKemp__Author).

Introduction

This book can save your relationship – and your sanity.

The menopause might happen to women – but it hits men, too. And if you've picked up this book, chances are you're already feeling the fallout: the moods, the mania, the mayhem.

Maybe you're wondering why she can't sleep. How a minor thing can spark a major meltdown. Or why she just burst into tears over an advert for cat food.

One moment she's the love of your life. The next? It's like she's been body-snatched by her hormones. You're starting to worry you're both going mad ... and slowly drifting apart.

Welcome to *Burning Up, Frozen Out* – the book you didn't know you needed until things got, well, a little too hot to handle.

This isn't just a guide – it's your personal playbook for going from wide-eyed passenger to confident co-pilot. In 12 straight-talking (and surprisingly interesting) chapters, we'll tell you everything you need to know about the menopause but were too afraid to ask.

Our goal? To help you understand what's really going on, so you can rebuild your relationship and face whatever comes next with confidence, clarity and control – all while keeping your sense of humour firmly intact.

Why did we write this book?

Because we needed it.

When the menopause exploded into our lives, we went looking for a no-nonsense guide to explain what the hell was happening. Something informed, practical and actually useful. We drew a blank. There were plenty of brilliant menopause books for women, but hardly anything that spoke to us – and nothing that showed men how to step up without ballsing it up.

So we got to work. We spent months talking to some of the most passionate and well-informed experts on the planet. And not just women's health specialists. We spoke to world-renowned doctors, psychologists, neuroscientists, dietitians, sports physiologists, leading authorities on sleep, stress, sex and relationships plus a former special forces operative and even a hostage negotiator.

Why go this far? To leave no stone unturned in getting you the advice you need to navigate the weird, wild – and sweat-inducing – world of the menopause.

She's not broken so doesn't need fixing

Before we go any further, there's something you *really* need to know: she may say she feels 'broken' but it isn't your job to try to 'fix' her.

So if you've been carrying the weight of the world on your shoulders wanting to make everything better, take a breath ... and let it go.

She doesn't want Superman. She needs calm, consistent, and compassionate support. That means understanding what's happening to the woman you love – or your mum, your sister, cousin or colleague – and being the person they can always count on when they need you most.

Our mission is simple: to give you the knowledge, tools and confidence to show up and be that steady presence, even when you've got no idea what to do. The person who's always on her side when she can't find her car keys, is melting from another hot flush or her sleep has vanished faster than last month's pay cheque.

You'll hear from women who've lived it and the men who've ridden the relationship rollercoaster with them. Some clung on by their fingernails. Others actually learned to enjoy the ride. They'll share what helped, what backfired, and what they wish they'd done differently – so you can avoid the same rookie mistakes.

So if you're feeling out of your depth – and want to help without making things worse – you've come to the right place.

From here on, we've got your back – so you can focus on having hers.

What's inside? Everything you never realized you needed to know.

Part 1: Knowledge (Chapters 1–4)

This is your crash course in what the hell's going on with her body, her brain and her hormones, so you can ditch the guesswork and start joining the dots.

Want more good news? You'll soon realize that none of this is her fault – or yours, for that matter – and start getting the straight answers to your growing list of head-scratching questions.

Here's another thing no one warns you about: it's not just her being put through the wringer. Your mood's low. Your mojo's gone. You've got a creeping sense that your life isn't heading the way you wanted. It's OK. You're not broken. Your hormones are shifting, too, and it turns out midlife men and women have far more in common than you think. Once you know what you're both dealing with, everything starts to make sense – and that's when it begins to get easier.

Part 2: Communication (Chapters 5–8)

You've now got the knowledge – time to do something with it. Start talking. The thought of casual chats about your feelings, fears and frustrations may seem terrifying right now, but once you know how to have the right conversations, in the right way, at the right time, the words – along with feelings of relief and reconnection – will start to flow.

Once you're talking to one another, you can then have deeper conversations with people who have the power to make a real difference. Because at some point, she may need to speak to a doctor. The problem? So many women get fobbed off or failed by medical professionals, so it's vital you know how to navigate the healthcare system together. You'll learn how to prepare for appointments, ask the right questions, and push for the support she deserves. We'll also cover the different treatments available – including hormone replacement therapy (HRT) – how they work, the potential pros and cons, and how she can weigh up what's right for her.

Part 3: Power (Chapters 9–12)

You know what's going on and how to talk about it. There's one final step: action. Because small steps can lead to big wins for your health, happiness and relationship.

We'll show you how to stress less, sleep deeper, eat better and move more – all with minimal time, fuss and effort – to help ease the worst of her symptoms. They'll also boost her mood, energy and confidence. The best bit? They'll work for you, too, and they won't just make a difference for the present situation. A few better habits now will set up both of you to live a longer, stronger and more fun-filled life.

And yes, we'll talk about sex, too, and how to bring back the intimacy, connection and spark, so your bond doesn't just survive this stage, but deepens, strengthens ... and lasts.

Flush vs flash: The UK–US hormone divide

A quick word on housekeeping (and heads-up: this won't be the last time we remind you about domestic duties). Ever wondered whether 'oestrogen' and 'estrogen' are different hormones? Or whether 'hot flash' is a classic menopause symptom or a straight-to-streaming Marvel superhero spin-off? Don't worry – it's not you, it's just the Atlantic divide.

We use British English in this book. Here's a quick cheat sheet so you don't get caught out:

> **Oestrogen vs estrogen:** Same hormone, different spelling. The UK sticks with its Greek roots; the US keeps it simple and sounds it out.
> **Hot flush vs hot flash:** British women flush, Americans flash. Either way, it's a sudden internal bonfire, often accompanied by a bucket load of sweat and a surge of anxiety.
> **HRT vs MHT:** The UK calls it hormone replacement therapy (HRT), the US prefers menopausal hormone therapy (MHT). Different names, same idea – topping up hormones to restore balance and ease symptoms.
> **GP vs OB-GYN:** In the UK, she'll see a GP (general practitioner). In the US, it's often an OB-GYN (pronounced *Oh-Bee-Gee-Why-En*). The difference? A GP is a jack-of-all-trades; an OB-GYN is a women's health mastermind.
> **Menopause vs the menopause:** Even the word 'menopause' divides us. In the UK, it's *the* menopause. In the US, just *menopause*. Like *the flu* vs *flu*. Drop the definitive article if you like – just don't drop the conversation.

A last word on our language – and your limitations

One last thing. In *Burning Up, Frozen Out*, we use terms like 'female', 'woman' and 'women' to refer to biological sex – people born with ovaries – unless otherwise stated. The same goes for 'male', 'man' and 'men' – we use these terms to mean people born with testes.

Also, this book is here to unpack how hormones and habits shape health, behaviour, mood, energy, and the way we relate to each other. It's here to inform – not diagnose – and definitely not to help you win an argument.

So read up – because the more you know, the more you can help your missus, mum, mate or colleague.

But no, don't ever say, 'You're a bit peri today,' over Sunday lunch just because someone burned the roast chicken. And if you catch yourself at a work meeting mansplaining the menopause off a single chart from Chapter 2? Shut the slideshow and sit back down.

Part 1
KNOWLEDGE

1

Your time to shine
How to be the everyday hero she needs

Let's begin with the elephant in the room: you've absolutely no idea what the hell is going on.

She didn't come with a manual, and you're pretty sure you didn't miss the memo. Yet here we are – she's snappy, she's sad, and she's not sleeping. All at the same time. And you're afraid to open your mouth in case you say the wrong thing – again.

Relax. You're in the right place. You'll soon know what menopause is, why it matters, and why you – yes, you – are the man who can make all the difference. And the good news keeps coming: you're also going to get hours of your life back from no longer being glued to Google, trying to figure out why her world's suddenly turned upside down.

The best bit? None of this is as bad as it might seem. So let's dial down the pressure. This isn't about fixing her, or saving her. It's about stepping up and showing her she's not in this alone.

In this chapter you'll discover:

- Why most women don't understand the menopause and why you're not supposed to either
- The three stages of menopause and what they actually mean for her (and for you)
- How to spot the early warning signs her hormones are going haywire
- Why so many relationships fall apart in midlife and how to stop yours becoming a statistic
- How menopause can change her behaviour and why taking it personally only makes things worse
- How to be the man who makes her life easier, not more overwhelming.

If you're reading this – whether you picked it up yourself, it magically appeared on your bedside table, or it was launched in your direction by the love of your life with a cry of, 'For the love of God, read this!' – then the menopause is either on the horizon or already here.

And while your instinct may be to hide in your man cave for the next decade until it all blows over, well, sorry, that's not going to cut it.

Most men today aren't like our fathers or grandfathers. We don't want to be silent bystanders in the defining moments of our partner's life, watching from the sidelines through pregnancy, parenthood and, now, perimenopause. (We'll explain the difference between perimenopause, menopause and postmenopause shortly.)

We want to show up. Step up. Play a real part.

The problem? Understanding the menopause can feel like the emotional equivalent of building an IKEA wardrobe, but with Japanese instructions, no Allen key, and both hands tied behind your back.

The good news? You don't need to figure it out alone, and with the right tools, you can build a rock-solid relationship.

Menopause 101

From peri to post – what each stage actually means

Perimenopause, menopause, postmenopause: if these terms are a bit fuzzy, you're not alone. One in four British men don't know what the menopause is, and only half believe they know someone who has experienced it.[1] Here's a quick topline on each stage, based on guidance from the British Menopause Society.[2] Don't worry – we're not going to test you, but we will go into more detail about the what, why and when in the next chapter.

Perimenopause is the hormonal build-up to menopause. It usually begins in a woman's forties and is when most of the common symptoms – hot flushes, brain fog, fatigue and anxiety – first appear. It can last for years. She can still get pregnant, even if her periods are all over the place.

Menopause means she hasn't had a period for 12 consecutive months. Her reproductive years are over – she can no longer get pregnant.

Postmenopause is everything after that. Her periods are done, but some symptoms – and long-term health risks – can stick around.

Menopause: One word – a billion different stories

Right now, around 13 million women in the UK are going through perimenopause or the menopause – that's roughly one-third of the country's entire female population.[3]

In the US, it's 75 million women, with around 6,000 more entering menopause every single day.[4]

And 2025 marked the moment when more than *one billion* women around the world were in perimenopause, menopause or postmenopause.[5]

Menopause can hit like a wrecking ball, or barely register at all. For many, it's a confusing, distressing and life-changing transition that can profoundly affect a woman's physical, mental and emotional health. An astonishing one in ten women report having suicidal thoughts during this time.[6]

But for others, it's not nearly so bad. In fact, up to one in five women report no symptoms at all.[7] And that's one of the trickiest things about this stage of life – no two women experience it the same.

How to spot the early warning signs

The first clues of perimenopause don't usually come with any fanfare. They sneak in – subtle, random and easy to ignore. That's why so many women shrug them off, blame stress or poor sleep, and struggle to join the dots back to their hormones. These are some of the more common early symptoms to watch for.[8] We'll get to all the obvious and obscure ones, and what causes them, in Chapter 2.

Brain fog: she's mid-sentence and forgets what she was saying – and she's lost her car keys, again

Acute anxiety: she's suddenly withdrawn, quiet or dodging social stuff she used to enjoy

Trouble sleeping: she can't fall asleep, stay asleep or wakes up at 4 AM wired and tired

Random rage: she blows her top over the tiniest thing, like the sound of your breathing

Aches and pains: she's started complaining about sore muscles and stiff joints, for no obvious reason

Low libido: she's gone off sex – and doesn't know why – and is more physically distant with you overall

Clueless? Confused? Of course she is

The average age of menopause is 51, but some women go through it much sooner. Around one in 100 experience it before 40 – what's known as premature menopause, or premature ovarian insufficiency – and around one in 1,000 before they even turn 30.[9] Early menopause, which happens between 40 and 45, affects about 10 percent of women.[10]

And while there's now a growing amount of research, advice and support for women going through the menopause, the majority are still massively underprepared. A UK government survey of almost 100,000 women found that 91 percent felt they didn't have enough information about the menopause, and more than a third didn't feel comfortable talking about it with a healthcare professional.[11]

Research from University College London found that just 2 percent of women felt well informed about the menopause before their symptoms began, and nearly two-thirds said they hadn't been informed at all.[12]

It's hardly a surprise. When do you think the menopause started being taught in British secondary schools? The late 1980s? The mid-1990s? Nope. September 2020.[13] Before that? Nothing. And many doctors are also in the dark – menopause training isn't mandatory, and most UK and US medical schools don't even cover it (see Chapter 7) – so they often miss the signs not only in their patients but in themselves (see Chapter 3).

> **Instant expert**
>
> **Dr Nicky Keay on how midlife hormones wreak havoc**
>
> *Dr Nicky Keay is a medical doctor, hormone specialist, and author of Myths of Menopause.[14] She's on a mission to help women take back control of their midlife health and happiness (nickykeayfitness.com).*
>
> Even as a woman with a medical background I felt like I was falling apart at times. You have to tell yourself that the menopause isn't a disease, it's a natural life stage. But without the right information, it can feel like you're falling apart. Seemingly unrelated symptoms can crop up, and if you don't know what's happening, it can feel overwhelming. But understanding what's going on – and knowing it's not an illness – gives you power. It helps you make practical decisions.

She didn't see it coming, so how could you?

If most women hit 40 with only a vague idea of what's coming,[15] and just one in five received any menopause education at school,[16] it's no wonder we men are completely in the dark, too – not just about what menopause really is but about the psychological and physical toll it can take. On her. And on us.

It's not that we don't care; it's that we've been left out of the conversation entirely. That's why we wrote this book: to help husbands, boyfriends, partners, sons, friends and colleagues first understand what the hell is going on, and then learn how to actually help.

Because menopause is a life-altering experience for everyone involved – not just the woman going through it. And many men describe this phase as a traumatic period of confusion, disconnection and suffering.[17] Communication collapses. Relationships break down. And too often, everyone ends up struggling alone, in silence.

Real talk

'My wife thought she was going to die – and so did I'

Rob Kemp is the co-author of this book and a freelance journalist who has written extensively about men's health, parenting and sport for more than 30 years. He's married to a long-suffering QPR fan, Amanda, and it was an incident at Loftus Road involving his wife that made his world stand still.

It was a phone call I'll never forget.

'I don't want to worry you, Rob, but we're just waiting for an ambulance to come for Amanda – she's having a problem with her heart.'

For months my wife had been experiencing bouts of anxiety, sleepless nights and worrying thoughts that she might die at any moment. We'd had a weekend away and she'd stayed up all night because she was worried that if she went to sleep she might not wake up. 'I'd sit on the train thinking I'm not going to get home because I'm going to have a heart attack,' she'd later tell me.

She went to her GP, who told her to cut back on the coffee. We didn't know what was causing this anxiety. The menopause never

> really came into the conversation because she wasn't experiencing the stereotypical symptoms.
>
> Then one Saturday afternoon, while she was at a football match with her parents, something she'd been doing for more than 40 years, her heart began racing – and not because QPR were playing like 1970s Brazil. Her mum took her home, called an ambulance and then phoned me.
>
> Following that incident and further consultations with her GP, it became clear that the anxiety, palpitations and sleepless nights were all symptoms of the menopause. At last we knew, at last she could get the treatment she needed to cope with what she was going through.

Why men need to know the truth

Here's a stat that should make every married man sit up: over 60 percent of divorces in the UK are initiated by women in their forties, fifties and sixties[18] – the exact time they're most likely to be dealing with huge hormonal changes – and 73 percent of women say the menopause played a role in the breakdown of their marriage.[19] That's not a coincidence. That's a crisis, and it's a similar picture across the pond.

'In the US, around 70 percent of divorces after the age of 30 are initiated by women,' says Dr Kelly Casperson, a urologist, author and podcast host who specializes in helping women – and their partners – better understand sex, desire and connection during midlife (kellycaspersonmd.com). 'Among educated women with advanced degrees, that figure jumps to 90 percent. That tells me men don't want to get divorced – but it's still happening, often around midlife.'[20]

Don't let the sun set on what matters most

Marriages often break down like that Ernest Hemingway line from *The Sun Also Rises* about how you go broke: *gradually, then suddenly*.

As Dr Casperson explains, emotional closeness gets replaced by frustration and silence. He wants sex to feel connected. She avoids it because it hurts, or because she feels exhausted, isolated or uncomfortable in her own skin. So they stop going to bed at the same time. Stop touching. Stop talking. And just when things feel at their most fragile, he might start dealing with midlife issues of his own – like rock-bottom mood, energy and motivation, or erectile dysfunction. And then, one day, they've drifted so far apart that there's no turning back.

'So if you're asking why men should care about menopause – this is it,' she says. 'If you want a happy relationship, want to feel loved and connected, and don't want to get divorced, you have to understand what's happening.'

You're not the problem, but you are part of the solution

Whether it's your partner, or your mum, your sister or your colleague, the menopause can shift the ground beneath a relationship. If you don't know what's going on, it's easy to get the wrong end of the stick – to take her mood swings personally, or mistake exhaustion and withdrawal for disinterest or rejection. You might think she's pulling away, when, in reality, she's running on empty. That gap in awareness is where frustration, miscommunication and emotional distance start creeping in.

'When men speak to me about the effect the menopause is having on their relationship, there's a pattern,' explains Diane Danzebrink, founder of UK-based Menopause Support (menopausesupport.co.uk) and author of *Making Menopause Matter*.[21] 'They don't understand why their partner appears to have changed – why she's become withdrawn, more anxious or emotional, less patient, less sociable, and lost interest in sex and intimacy. The words these men use to describe how they feel? Confused, worried, isolated and lonely.'

The good news? This doesn't have to be a breaking point. It can be a turning point.

As you'll discover in this book, understanding what's actually going on, being able to talk about it together, and offering practical support can not only help you stay together but also help you come out stronger. And the men who learn to understand the menopause aren't just helping their partner, they're helping themselves, and every relationship they care about.

> ### Instant expert
>
> **Kathy Abernethy on cutting through menopause misinformation**
>
> *Kathy Abernethy is a trustee of the British Menopause Society, a registered menopause specialist, and author of* Menopause: The one-stop guide.[22] *She's a firm believer that the right support can change everything, if you know where to find it (kathyabernethy.com).*
>
> **Don't assume you know what she's up against**
> People think menopause is short, natural and no big deal. It can be anything but. Some women sail through it, yes, but others are hit hard, and it can happen earlier than you think. The truth? Every experience is different, and a lot of what you think you know may be wrong.
>
> **Check your sources**
> Be curious, but be careful. There's a lot of misinformation out there, especially online. If someone's selling something, check whether it's backed by evidence. Does it align with the National Institute for Health and Care Excellence (NICE) guidelines? The gold standard is consistency across credible sources – that's your clue it's trustworthy.
>
> **Don't believe everything you read on the internet**
> Online and social media support groups can be helpful, but some are full of dodgy advice and scare stories. Take it all with a pinch of salt and cross-check anything that sounds off. Misinformation causes fear, and right now, she doesn't need more of that.

This is where things start to make sense

So now you know: you're not supposed to have all the answers. You're not falling short. You've just never been told what's really going on – until now.

You've already done the most important thing by showing up. Because when you understand what she's going through – and why it's happening – you can stop reacting and start responding. That's when everything starts to change, for the better.

In the next chapter, we'll dive into what's actually going on inside her body. Buckle up, we're heading into hormone territory. And yes, it might sound complicated, but once you know a bit of the science, all the chaos starts to make a lot more sense.

2

What the hell is happening?
Welcome to the hormone horror show

Now you know she's not losing her mind – it's her hormones staging a take-no-prisoners mutiny.

This chapter explains what's really happening to her brain and body. But don't worry – this isn't a boring biology lesson. It's your access-all-areas pass to what's really going on behind the scenes. You'll meet the hormonal heavyweights, find out what happens when they go rogue, and finally get your head around why everything feels so chaotic, confusing ... and totally out of control.

In this chapter you'll discover:

- The four stages of her menopause journey and how to tell where she is now
- Why perimenopause is the real hormonal storm, not menopause itself
- What hormones actually are and what happens when they go haywire
- How oestrogen, progesterone and testosterone shape her health, mood and motivation
- The five hard-hitting symptoms to spot on your radar – from brain fog to vanishing libido
- Why no two women go through menopause the same way, and what that means for you.

Let's get one thing straight: this is not your fault.

Yes, she's flinching every time you get too close. She's swearing like a sailor because someone's 'moved' her car keys. And she's crying her heart out at an episode of *MasterChef* like it's the closing scene of *Marley & Me*.

But it's not really about you – or actually about anything. It's her hormones.

They're spiking, crashing, vanishing – and behaving like teenagers home alone for the weekend: no control, no conscience, and absolutely no intention of sticking around to clean up the mess or face any of the consequences.

Hormones gone haywire: A beginner's guide

Luckily, you don't need a medical degree to understand how hormones work or the havoc they can cause. A little knowledge goes a long way. Once you've got your head around what hormones do, and what happens when they go rogue, things start to make a lot more sense.

So what are hormones, exactly? They're chemical messengers – think of them as your body's push notifications: a steady stream of updates, instructions and alerts between glands, organs, tissues and cells, keeping everything running smoothly. They control everything: energy, sleep, sex drive, temperature, emotions, digestion – in short, the entire operating system.[1]

It's not as complicated as it sounds, but if you're thinking, 'It's all Greek to me', you're actually spot on. The word 'hormone' comes from the Greek *hormō*, meaning 'to excite or arouse'. And while we're here, menopause – meaning the end of her menstrual cycle – comes from the Greek words *men* (month) and *pausis* (pause).

That's your language lesson done. Now, it's time for chemistry – and the chaos.

The chemical culprits behind the chaos

Three key hormones – often referred to as the sex hormones – help keep her mind, body and everything else ticking along nicely: oestrogen, progesterone and testosterone. The first two are the leading ladies of the female reproductive system. From embryo onwards, they call the shots – shaping her into a woman, kicking off puberty, running the menstrual cycle, and juggling everything from mood to metabolism. For us, testosterone is the main man. It's what makes us male – telling our bodies to grow beards and biceps, and our brains to be confident, motivated and horny.

But women produce testosterone, too – just in smaller amounts, like we do with oestrogen[2] – quietly working behind the scenes, fuelling energy, assertiveness and sexual desire.

Recurring roles: Enter the ensemble

Other hormones also play a role in her health, fertility and daily life, but they're more supporting cast than lead characters. Follicle-stimulating hormone (FSH) and luteinizing hormone (LH) help regulate her menstrual cycle.[3] Cortisol controls stress,[4] melatonin influences sleep,[5] and insulin manages energy, blood sugar and weight.[6]

For most of her teens, twenties and thirties, these hormones work in harmony. Then perimenopause rocks up and rips up the script. Oestrogen and progesterone become total divas – one minute demanding all the attention, the next vanishing without a trace – and the fallout can be fierce.

The ensemble cast panic: FSH and LH surge to get the ovaries back on track,[7] cortisol spikes,[8] melatonin falters[9] and insulin sensitivity tanks[10] – and the chaos really kicks in.

Here's a closer look at the intended role of the three main players and what happens when they completely lose the plot.

Oestrogen

How to say it: EE-struh-jen (UK), ESS-truh-jin (US)

Impact: 10/10. The A-list star of the show

What it does: Keeps her cool, calm, collected and every one of her systems firing. It protects her bones, balances her mood, boosts her libido, supports sleep, makes sex feel good and so much more.[11] It's basically the Swiss Army knife of hormones.

What happens: Oestrogen levels swing wildly, then drop like a stone. Cue hot flushes, brain fog, mood crashes, vaginal dryness, poor sleep, creaky joints, plus many more physical and mental health problems.[12]

Treatment options: Hormone replacement therapy (usually as patches, gels or pills) can help top up oestrogen and bring many symptoms back under control (see Chapter 8).[13]

Progesterone

How to say it: pruh-JESS-ter-own (UK), pro-JESS-ter-own (US)

Impact: 8/10. The behind-the-scenes talent that keeps the show running smoothly

What it does: Acts as her internal calming system – keeping oestrogen in check, stabilizing mood, supporting sleep, regulating periods and protecting the womb.[14] It's not glamorous, but it's the glue that keeps things together.

What happens: Levels crash first and fast. This throws everything off balance, often triggering anxiety, mood swings, irritability, restless sleep and irregular periods.

Treatment options: Often combined with oestrogen in HRT, especially if she still has her uterus. It protects the womb lining and helps restore hormonal balance.

Testosterone

How to say it: tes-TOSS-ter-own (UK/US)

Impact: 6/10. The minor character you only miss when they're gone

What it does: Yes, women have testosterone, too. It drives her desire – for sex, but also for life. Supports mood, motivation, muscle tone, energy, focus and overall health.[15]

What happens: Levels decline steadily from her twenties, and then tank in midlife. That can mean lower libido, flat mood, fatigue, and a sense she's lost her purpose. It's like her spark's gone out – and she's run out of matches.

Treatment options: Some women benefit from testosterone therapy to improve sex drive, energy and mood. It's not officially licensed for women, but under NICE guidelines, it can be prescribed off-label for low sexual desire when HRT alone isn't enough and other causes have been ruled out (see Chapter 8).[16]

Her hormone heatmap

From puberty to postmenopause

Here's how oestrogen, progesterone and testosterone levels change across a woman's life.

Oestrogen and progesterone rise at puberty, then fluctuate in monthly cycles during the reproductive years. In perimenopause, their levels become more erratic and start to decline. After menopause, both hormones remain low and stable for the rest of her life.[17]

Testosterone also increases during puberty, peaks in the early twenties, and then declines gradually and steadily with age.[18]

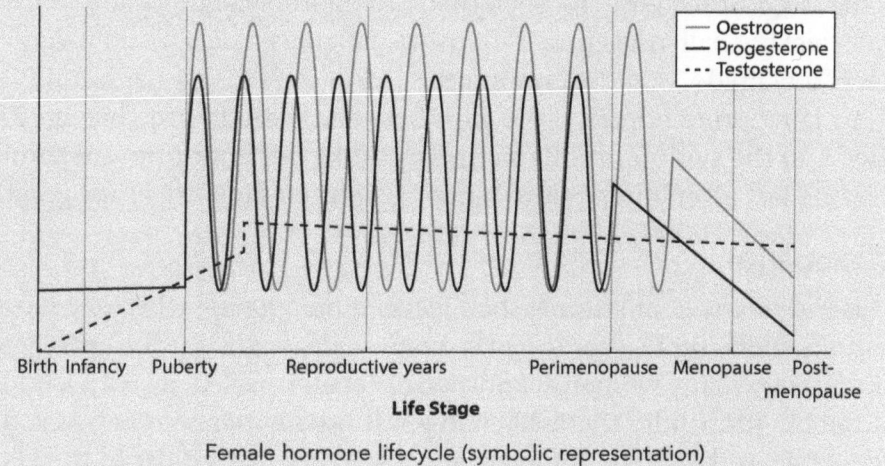

Female hormone lifecycle (symbolic representation)

Four acts – one hell of a plot twist

You've met the main players – oestrogen, progesterone and testosterone – but to really understand what's going on, you need to see how their character arc unfolds over time.

Here's a quick outline of the four hormonal acts of her life – premenopause, perimenopause, menopause and postmenopause – so you can figure out where she is, what's going on and what's coming next.

Premenopause

This is the hormonal 'normal' – her reproductive years, from puberty until perimenopause. Each month, she's ovulating, menstruating and can get pregnant. Oestrogen and progesterone follow a (mostly) predictable pattern, and any symptoms are usually chalked up to premenstrual syndrome (PMS) – which affects over 90 percent of women, often with headaches, bloating and the occasional spot you can see from the International Space Station.[19] She may also rip your clothes off, depending where she is in her cycle. So far, so good.

Perimenopause

This is the bumpy and often bewildering prelude to menopause, and it can last for years. It usually kicks off in her mid-forties, though for some women, the changes begin in their late thirties. At first, things just feel a bit off: periods become erratic – they show up late, overstay their welcome or ghost her entirely. Then oestrogen starts swinging like a hormonal wrecking ball, triggering hot flushes, fatigue, anxiety, brain fog, poor sleep, low libido, and the creeping suspicion she's losing her mind.[20]

In late perimenopause, the gaps between periods stretch even further, and the symptoms often ramp up – like her hormones are throwing one last all-nighter before hanging up their glow sticks for good.[21]

Menopause

This is the official milestone: she's reached menopause when she hasn't had a period for 12 months in a row[22] – although it's not exactly an anniversary many women acknowledge, let alone celebrate with a bottle of bubbly (hopefully that will change). It usually happens between the ages of 45 and 55 – the UK average is 51,[23] and a year older in the US.[24]

It means her ovaries have officially downed tools, oestrogen levels have plateaued, and she can no longer get pregnant. But menopause isn't really a single moment, and the symptoms don't politely pack up just because her periods have.[25]

Postmenopause

This is everything that comes after. It starts one year after her final period and carries on for the rest of her life. With average female life expectancy now well into the eighties across the Western world, she could spend around a third of her life in this stage. Some symptoms settle down. Others are like Wile E. Coyote – stubborn, steadfast and with no intention of ever calling it a day. Even if the hormonal chaos has eased, the long-term effects of low oestrogen – on her bones, brain and heart – are still unfolding.[26]

> ### Real talk
>
> **'One week every month I feel like I'm going crazy'**
>
> *I'm Caitlin. I'm 42, live in New York City with my husband and our three kids, and work as a writer, podcaster and content strategist. I also spend a lot of time shouting into the internet about motherhood, mental health and midlife – mostly so other women know they're not alone (bigtimeadulting.blog).*
>
> My perimenopause symptoms began around age 38, after having my third child. Before kids, my monthly cycle was basically a non-event – no real PMS, no cramps, just very minor symptoms. But now, the week before my period feels like 'hell week'. I get really anxious and down, I'm irritable, and little things – like my kids or my husband – can drive me crazy. Physically, I'm now experiencing bloating, cramps, headaches and even night sweats some nights, none of which I had before children.
>
> One of the hardest parts is the uncertainty. I don't know how much worse my symptoms might get or how long they'll last. My mother and grandmother went through menopause early, so I wonder if that will happen to me, too, but nobody can say for sure. The unpredictability can be really anxiety-inducing. The best I can do is remind myself this isn't my fault – it's hormonal – and try to be kinder to myself. Also, talking openly with friends really helps. We're all going through something similar, even if our experiences differ. It helps us feel less alone. As for my husband? There's not a whole lot he can do – beyond the fact that he believes me and is understanding of my fluctuating hormones. We also use humour to defuse tension around my tension, which always helps.

When her hormones don't follow the script

Not every woman follows the classic four-act menopause. For some, the curtain falls far earlier than expected – or drops without warning. These experiences are rare, but often more disruptive, more dramatic and more traumatic – which is exactly why they deserve just as much attention.

Early menopause

If she hasn't had a period for 12 consecutive months between the ages of 40 and 45, it's considered early menopause.[27] The symptoms are the same, but they start much younger, often catching women off guard. It might come on by itself or be brought about by an underlying health condition. And while it's not something many people talk about, it affects around 1 in 20 women.[28]

Premature menopause

In some cases, menopause arrives far earlier than expected – before a woman turns 40. This is known as premature menopause and can be caused by inherited factors, certain illnesses, or medical treatments like chemotherapy that affect the ovaries.[29] It's rare, affecting about 1 in 100 women,[30] but the impact can be brutal: sudden fertility loss, intense symptoms, and a deep sense of grief for the life stage that ended too soon.

Surgical menopause

When both ovaries are surgically removed – typically during a hysterectomy or as part of cancer treatment – it causes a sudden, severe and permanent drop in hormones. There's no gradual build-up, just an instant shift into full-blown menopause.[31] Symptoms can be intense and fast, which is why it's sometimes called 'crash' or 'sudden' menopause (see Chapter 7).

Oestrogen 101

It's not just about periods and pregnancy

Oestrogen plays a key role in fertility and the menstrual cycle. That's why, when levels drop and the ovaries stop releasing eggs, her periods stop and natural pregnancy is no longer possible.

But why does falling oestrogen affect so much more than just reproduction?

Because the obvious symptoms of perimenopause – anxiety, insomnia, brain fog, hot flushes, digestive issues, joint pain – are just the beginning. Over time, low oestrogen also raises her risk of dementia, heart disease, osteoporosis, muscle loss, weight gain, insulin resistance and type-2 diabetes.[32] How can one hormone do all that?

Oestrogen: Everywhere, all at once

Oestrogen isn't just about periods and pregnancy. It's a whole-body hormone, with receptors almost everywhere – in the brain, gut, heart, skin, muscles and more.[33] It helps regulate everything from temperature and

What the hell is happening?

mood to memory and metabolism.[34] So when levels fall during perimenopause and menopause, the effects are widespread and often overwhelming.

Here's how oestrogen keeps everything working in harmony and why its absence is felt everywhere:

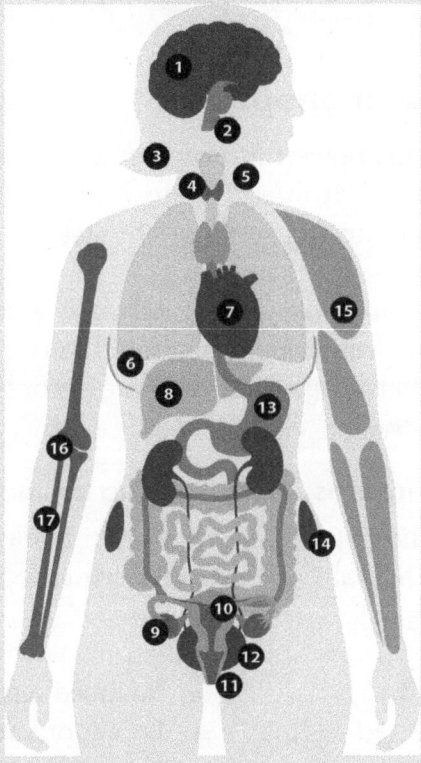

1 *Brain:* Boosts memory, focus and mood
2 *Brainstem:* Regulates sleep and temperature
3 *Skin and Hair:* Maintains collagen, hydration and growth
4 *Thyroid:* Influences metabolism and energy balance
5 *Immune system:* Supports response and lowers inflammation
6 *Breasts:* Shapes tissue and density
7 *Heart:* Protects blood vessels and lowers cholesterol
8 *Liver:* Regulates cholesterol and blood sugar
9 *Ovaries:* Regulates egg development and release
10 *Uterus:* Controls the menstrual cycle and womb lining
11 *Vagina:* Keeps tissue moist, elastic and healthy
12 *Bladder:* Maintains tissue tone and control

> 13 *Gut:* Supports digestion and gut health
> 14 *Fat tissue:* Regulates storage and distribution
> 15 *Muscles:* Maintains strength and power
> 16 *Joints:* Improves movement and reduces stiffness
> 17 *Bones:* Preserves strength and density

The signs of perimenopause

When a hormone this powerful drops off a cliff, it doesn't just affect one part of her body – it affects almost all of them. From acne to anxiety, bloating to brain fog, and sketchy sleep to scratchy skin – the fallout can be relentless and confusing.

Some symptoms are physical. Others are emotional or mental. A few are just plain weird. But they're all very real, and for many women, they're exhausting. Here they are – confusing, chaotic, but completely normal.[35]

Psychological symptoms: What's going on in her head?

Here are some of the cognitive, emotional, behavioural and neurological symptoms that can occur from perimenopause onwards.

Behavioural and social

- Social withdrawal
- Feeling disconnected or not like herself
- Increased sensitivity to stress
- Loss of self-esteem
- Reduced resilience
- Low motivation
- New or increased health anxiety
- Difficulty coping with workload or routine tasks

Cognitive and mental function

- Brain fog
- Poor concentration
- Memory problems
- Difficulty finding words
- Indecisiveness
- Clumsiness
- Loss of coordination
- Disorientation
- Difficulty navigating familiar places

Emotional and mood

- Low mood
- Anxiety
- Irritability
- Mood swings
- Tearfulness
- Panic attacks
- Surges of unexpected emotion
- Anger or rage episodes
- Feeling flat or emotionally numb
- Loss of confidence
- Loss of interests, hobbies or passions

> **Perimenopause: Plain sailing or perfect storm?**
>
> About one in four women sail through perimenopause with few or no symptoms.[36] At the other extreme, around 10 percent have suicidal thoughts due to the severity of their experience.[37] Proof, if ever it was needed, that no two menopause journeys are the same and that some are unimaginably harder than others.

Physical symptoms: What's going on in her body?

And now for the rest of the symptom circus: the sensory, metabolic, hormonal and just plain weird.

Reproductive and sexual

- Irregular periods
- Heavy periods
- Lighter or skipped periods
- Changes in menstrual cycle length
- Vaginal dryness
- Painful or inflamed vulva
- Painful sex
- Low or fluctuating libido
- UTIs

Metabolic and energy

- Fatigue or low energy
- Blood sugar crashes
- Shakiness between meals
- Weight gain around the tummy
- Body fat redistribution
- Food cravings
- Palpitations
- Feeling cold all the time
- Sudden fluctuations in body temperature

Muscles and joints

- Joint pain or stiffness
- Frozen shoulder
- Plantar fasciitis
- Muscle aches or weakness
- Restless legs
- Tingling or numbness in hands and feet

Skin, hair and senses

- Sensitivity to noise or light
- Dry, itchy or sensitive skin
- Acne or skin changes
- Body odour changes
- Changes to sense of smell
- Changes to nail strength or growth
- Thinning hair
- Increased facial hair
- Loss of eyebrow or eyelash density
- Dry eyes
- Itchy ears
- Tinnitus
- Electric shock sensations
- Increased thirst
- Dry mouth
- Gum problems or bleeding gums
- Burning mouth or tongue

Sleep and recovery

- Insomnia and sleep disruption
- Restless sleep
- Multiple wake-ups
- Waking too early
- Night sweats

Other physical symptoms

- Hot flushes
- Bloating
- Digestive changes
- Constipation
- Diarrhoea
- New or worsening allergies or intolerances
- Urinary urgency or incontinence
- More colds or infections
- Worsening of existing autoimmune conditions

Symptom spotlight: 5 problems that can hit her for six

Every woman's experience is unique – but some symptoms are repeat offenders. Here are five of the most common, confusing or crippling signs of perimenopause, and what's causing them. Don't worry about doing anything to help just yet – we'll get to that in a bit.

Symptom spotlight #1 – Hot flushes and night sweats

How many women get it? About 70 percent.[38]

What does it feel like? Hot flushes are sudden, intense waves of heat that spread across the face, neck and chest, often followed by sweating, blushing and a pounding heart. Each one typically lasts between one and five minutes,[39] but the after-effects, like chills or fatigue, can linger for longer. Some women get a few a week. Others get them every hour.[40] Night sweats are episodes of excessive sweating that wreck sleep, kill intimacy, spark fury, and have her tossing, turning and melting for hours.

What causes them? Hot flushes and night sweats are both vasomotor symptoms, caused by falling oestrogen disrupting the brain's internal thermostat.[41] It starts overreacting to even minor changes in body temperature as if she's overheating, and responds by widening blood vessels and triggering sweating and flushing to cool her down.

What makes it worse? Spicy food, alcohol, caffeine, stress and overheating caused by, for example, a stuffy bedroom or thick pyjamas.[42] Being overweight or obese makes them more likely and more severe, as does smoking.[43]

What helps? HRT is the gold standard,[44] and other non-hormonal medications – including certain antidepressants – are also approved (see Chapter 8).[45] Simple habit changes can make a difference, too: cutting out common triggers, losing weight, stopping smoking, dressing in layers, keeping the bedroom cool, and – for some – cognitive behavioural therapy (CBT).[46]

Symptom spotlight #2 – Brain fog

How many women get it? Around 73 percent.[47]

What does it feel like? She goes blank mid-sentence, forgets why she walked into a room, and can't remember names, plans or passwords. She might laugh it off at first – until the lapses stop being funny and start feeling like her brain's on dodgy Wi-Fi, cutting out every time she tries to think straight.

What causes it? Oestrogen helps regulate key neurotransmitters involved in focus and memory. As levels fluctuate, it can feel like her brain is constantly buffering.[48]

What makes it worse? Multitasking, sleep deprivation, stress and too much coffee. Feeling embarrassed or judged can also knock her confidence and thicken the fog.

What helps? Regular exercise, better sleep, stress reduction,[49] and – for some women – hormone replacement therapy.[50] For many, just knowing it's hormonal can ease any fears that it's early dementia.

Symptom spotlight #3 – Anxiety and panic attacks

How many women get it? Around 69 percent.[51]

What does it feel like? Frantic thoughts, irrational fear, spiralling worry or overwhelming dread, often with chest tightness, breathlessness or a racing heart.[52] It can feel like something's seriously wrong – even like she's dying – and appear out of the blue, even if she's never had a panic attack before. It's the brain's way of going straight to DEFCON 1, even though it's a false alarm.

What causes it? Oestrogen and progesterone help regulate mood and calm the nervous system. When they drop, cortisol – the main stress hormone – can take over.[53]

What makes it worse? Stress, poor sleep, caffeine, alcohol and sudden hormonal dips – especially in the days before her period. Feeling unsupported can amplify it all.[54]

What helps? Stress-management strategies like exercise, mindfulness or breathing techniques, fewer stimulants, better sleep, HRT and therapy. And knowing it's hormonal can make a huge difference.

Symptom spotlight #4 – Disrupted sleep

How many women get it? About 84 percent.[55]

What does it feel like? She can't fall asleep, can't stay asleep, or wakes up at 3 AM wired but tired, like she's necked half a dozen vodka Red Bulls. Even the little sleep she does get is restless – so tomorrow will feel like an all-day hangover but without having had happy hour.

What causes it? Fluctuating oestrogen and progesterone affect production of melatonin – the hormone that promotes sleepiness – and disrupt the body's temperature control and stress response.[56] Stress and anxiety add to the pile-on.[57]

What makes it worse? Alcohol, caffeine, big evening meals and late-night doomscrolling.[58] And lying next to a snoring partner who could sleep through a Taylor Swift concert really rubs it in.

What makes it better? Consistent bed and wake-up times, a regular wind-down routine, a cool, dark and quiet bedroom,[59] reducing stress,[60] regular exercise,[61] and cognitive behavioural therapy for insomnia (CBT-I, see Chapter 9).[62] If symptoms are severe – especially when driven by hot flushes – HRT is often the most effective option.[63]

Symptom spotlight #5 – Painful vagina and low libido

How many women get it? About 40 percent experience vaginal problems or discomfort, and just over one in two report a loss of interest in sex.[64]

What does it feel like? There might be itching, dryness, soreness, or a sense that things just aren't right down there. Urinary tract infections (UTIs) become more common, and libido can drop off a cliff – sex may feel uncomfortable at best and excruciating at worst. Not exactly a recipe for romance, huh?

What causes it? Falling oestrogen causes thinning of the vaginal lining, reduced lubrication, and less blood flow 'downstairs'.[65] Low testosterone can also kill desire.[66]

What makes it worse? Physically: friction during sex can cause microtears in the vaginal tissue. Lack of arousal, poor lubrication, and certain soaps or washes can also increase irritation.[67] Emotionally: shame, silence, poor communication, and avoiding intimacy altogether can turn a treat into a trigger.[68] Feeling anxious, unattractive or misunderstood only widens the gap.

What helps? HRT[69] or vaginal oestrogen – which comes as a cream, pessary or ring – can work wonders.[70] Because it's applied locally, it's safe for most women, even those who can't take HRT. Testosterone can help boost libido, too,[71] if she can get it prescribed (see Chapter 8).

Instant expert

Dr Victoria Felkar on making sense of the hormonal hellscape

Dr Victoria Felkar, PhD, is a researcher and educator who specializes in how health, performance, hormones and modern life collide. Her work explores how hormones are shaped by different factors like sleep, stress, training, trauma, diet, culture and society – and why hormonal health should never be evaluated in isolation (victoriafelkar.com).

Hormones never work solo

Nothing in the body happens in isolation – it's a beautiful, chaotic dance. So it's not helpful to think of hormones as separate levers you can pull one at a time – they're a tangled web. If one goes off-key, the rest scramble to rebalance. When oestrogen dips, it 'talks' to cortisol, insulin, testosterone, thyroid hormones and other biochemicals, and systems of the body – the whole gang. That's why symptoms can feel random, intense and all over the place. And because this orchestra responds to everything – stress, illness, identity shifts, relationships, work – you need to see the full symphony, not chase one untuned instrument.

Every woman is unique, so expect the unexpected

There's no textbook perimenopause, just like there's no guaranteed 28-day menstrual cycle. Everyone starts perimenopause from a different hormonal baseline. One woman might breeze through; another might feel like her system is completely 'rewiring'. Change isn't linear or predictable. It's a kaleidoscope of individual baselines, life histories and environmental triggers. So when hormones begin to wobble, expect a few surprises.

She's not herself – and she knows it

Fluctuating hormone levels can make thoughts, moods and even physical sensations feel alien. If she's battling sleep problems, brain fog or sudden swells of emotion, it's not just in her head – it's her physiology in flux. What you see on the outside only hints at the storm inside, and that 'chaotic dance' can leave her feeling disconnected from everyone, even herself.

Her body's not breaking – it's recalibrating

Menopause isn't the end. It's a radical transition as her body stops being able to rely on ovarian hormones to support various biological functions. To keep things working, her body may look to other hormones, biochemicals and organs for help. If she's already under pressure, this shift can feel brutal, but it isn't a breakdown, it's adaptation – a systemic 'rebalancing act'. With the right support, this radical transition becomes a retuning, and she can start to feel like her old self again.

Now you know what you're up against

Let's not sugar-coat it: her mind and body are in total meltdown. Her control panel's lit up like a Christmas tree, the autopilot's gone AWOL, and she's flying blind through a storm with no co-pilot, no map, and no idea why the cockpit's on fire.

One minute she's overheating, the next she's in tears, then wide awake at 3 AM wondering if she's dying. She may have absolutely no idea what's going on.

Thankfully, you now do.

The hormonal havoc. The system update. The reasons why she feels like a stranger in her own skin. This isn't just a phase. It's a full-body reboot – physical, mental, emotional, relational – and no two women experience it the same.

Now it's time to take your knowledge into the wild. Because even if she hasn't realized what's up, her body is leaving clues.

If you're paying attention – and know what to look for – you'll start seeing her symptoms for what they really are: not problems to fix, but dots to join. Then it all starts to fall into place, and the real breakthroughs can begin.

3

Is it getting hot in here?
Spotting the signs before she does

You might know some of the symptoms, but can you spot them in the wild? This chapter hands you the cheat sheet: the early warning signs, the classic clues and the bizarre curveballs that don't make sense – until you realize what's behind them.

Because perimenopause doesn't kick the door down. It sneaks in. One forgotten word. One slammed door. One sleepless night at a time.

So if you're feeling confused, shut out or like something's changed but you didn't get the memo, you're not alone. Even many experts missed their own symptoms.

This chapter helps you piece it all together. You'll learn how to spot the signs, understand what's going on, reframe your reactions to make things better, not worse. And along the way, you might realize something else: she's not the only one struggling with some midlife mayhem – you really are in this together.

In this chapter you'll discover:

- Why even many experts don't recognize their own perimenopause until it's in full swing
- How to decode the everyday signs – from brain fog to energy crashes to food aisle freak-outs
- What's really going on when she's distant, sad, irritable – or even smells different
- The ten big mistakes most men make, and how to handle blow-ups like a Tibetan monk
- What not to say when she's spiralling and what to do instead
- Why midlife isn't just her crisis and the reasons you might need a little TLC, too.

First things first: if you're kicking yourself for not spotting the signs of perimenopause sooner, stop. You're not a women's health expert.

In fact, we'd wager that, until you picked up this book, all you really knew about that world was how to belt out the *Bodyform* jingle, or that tampons gave women in white jeans the power to do cartwheels on the beach.

You are clued up? There's still a good chance you missed – or misread – at least some of the signs.

How can we be so sure? Because almost every woman we spoke to for this book – including world-class doctors, campaigners and champions for women's health – failed to recognize perimenopause in themselves.

These are people who live and breathe this stuff. And still, they brushed off their symptoms as tiredness, stress, overwork, or believed it was something far more serious.

So if it blindsided you and your partner? You're far from alone. You're in excellent company, and we've got the confessions to prove it.

Missed the signs? So does everyone

If two of the UK's highest-profile menopause experts – women who've spent years researching, writing about or treating perimenopause – didn't identify it in themselves, then what chance do the rest of us have? Here are their stories.

Dr Louise Newson is a GP, best-selling author,[1] and the founder of both Newson Health Menopause and Wellbeing Centre, one of the UK's leading private menopause clinics, and Balance, a menopause education, support and tracking platform (drlouisenewson.co.uk).

> I was having night sweats. I'm not a sweaty person – but I'd be covered in sweat thinking, 'Lymphoma is a type of cancer that gives you night sweats. Maybe I've got that.' I was tired, my migraines were worse, but I was also setting up the clinic, setting up a website. When your brain doesn't function properly, so much brain energy is spent on immediate things like 'God, how am I gonna find my car keys?' or 'How am I gonna get to work in time?' You don't have the capacity to see the bigger picture.

Kate Muir is a journalist, campaigner and author of *Everything You Need to Know about the Menopause (But Were Too Afraid to Ask)*.[2] She wrote and produced *Sex, Myths and the Menopause* with Davina McCall, the Channel 4 documentary that helped shift the national conversation around HRT and menopause care (katemuir.co.uk).

'I was the film critic at *The Times* and I was losing my memory. I kept thinking, "I've forgotten the name of that film." But I was remembering 350 films a year, so maybe that's normal. Then one Saturday I was at home writing a shopping list and thought, "I must shave my legs." I wrote down the word "shaver". And I just sat there thinking – there is a better word for that thing than "shaver". It took me 15 minutes to remember it was "razor". And then I panicked because I thought I had Alzheimer's – my mum had died of Alzheimer's the year before.'

Midlife doesn't come with a manual

That's just one of the many strange things about perimenopause – it's happening to her, but she might not be the first person to notice.

Mood swings. Trouble sleeping. Complaints of tinnitus, a dry mouth, or the sensation of bugs crawling under her skin. And those are just a few of the typical – and some of the downright weird – signs she might be perimenopausal.

It's no wonder she might think she's losing the plot. But joining the dots is unbelievably hard. And that's a huge part of the problem.

As a man, it's reasonable to assume that a life stage this significant would come with proper education and support. That there'd be clear guidance. Checklists. Resources. A roadmap. A safety net. A system.

You'd be wrong.

Sex hormones 101

The five key players behind the mayhem

Here's a quick refresher on what her key hormones do, why they matter, and how they shape her health, mood and motivation:[3]

Oestrogen: The headline act. Regulates periods, mood, sleep, temperature, memory, skin, bones and sex drive. When it drops, so does almost everything – including resilience, energy and emotional stability.
Progesterone: The calming influence. Balances oestrogen, supports sleep and helps regulate cycles. It's one of the first to fall during perimenopause, which can crank up anxiety, irritability and insomnia.
Testosterone: Not just a man thing. Women make it, too, and it fuels libido, confidence, motivation and muscle mass.

> **Luteinizing hormone (LH):** Tells the ovaries to release an egg. As ovulation slows, LH levels spike, which can mess with mood, sleep and hormonal balance.
> **Follicle-stimulating hormone (FSH):** Stimulates the follicles that produce oestrogen. When the ovaries stop responding, FSH levels surge – a key sign that perimenopause is under way.

The cost of carrying this alone

Most women aren't given the tools, language or space to make sense of what's happening to them.[4] So they soldier on, thinking they're just burned out, overwhelmed or – like Dr Newson and Kate Muir – seriously ill.

And that's not the only reason things get missed. Some women admit they were in denial. Others internalize the social stigma and outdated cultural baggage that menopause marks the end of their 'worth'.[5] That they're no longer fertile, no longer sexual,[6] no longer ... visible. These are heavy thoughts to carry. And harder still to say out loud.

Until someone joins the dots, she's going to keep struggling – often in silence. And the consequences can be serious.[7] Women aged 50–54 have the highest suicide rate of any female age group in England and Wales, with 9.2 deaths per 100,000 people, according to recent data from the Office for National Statistics.[8] And nearly 8 percent of perimenopausal women have suicidal thoughts, compared to just 1 percent of women before or after menopause.

The stakes couldn't be higher.

> **Menopause and marital breakdown**
>
> Nearly three in four midlife women said menopause was a contributing factor in the breakdown of their marriage, and 67 percent said their symptoms led to increased arguments or incidents of domestic abuse within their relationship, according to a survey of more than 1,000 women by the Family Law Menopause Project and Newson Health.[9]

Eyes open, mouth closed

Despite the stakes, your job is surprisingly simple. You're not there to diagnose her. Or 'fix' her. And you certainly don't need to charge in guns blazing, waving this book in the air and shouting, 'I know what's wrong with you!'

No, your job is this: to pay closer attention. To notice what's changed. To spot what she might miss. To step back and see the full picture – not just the tears, the fear, the anger or the silence.

It means keeping an eye out for the common signs – and the bizarre ones – so you can start to piece it all together. It might be perimenopause. It might be something else. But it's definitely not nothing. Whatever it is, you'll be better equipped to offer the support, care and understanding she really needs.

Spotting the symptoms

A hot flush might be the most recognizable symptom of perimenopause, but it's not necessarily the most common. Fatigue, sleep problems and mood changes are just as likely[10] – and, in some studies, even more prevalent.[11]

That matters, because perimenopause is easy to miss or misread – by you, by her and even by healthcare professionals – especially if she's not experiencing the so-called 'classic' signs.

We covered many of them in the previous chapter, but here's a quick refresher on the most common – and the most surprising – symptoms, so you can fine-tune your antennae to spot any changes sooner.

Most common perimenopause symptoms (by percentage of women affected)	Most surprising perimenopause symptoms (by percentage of women affected)
Brain fog (90%)	Joint pain (34%)
Anxiety (86%)	Dry eyes (26%)
Fatigue (82%)	Heart palpitations (25%)
Memory problems (80%)	Hair dryness/thinning (20%)
Sleep problems (79%)	Tinnitus (19%)
Low mood (79%)	Weight gain (18%)
Low libido (78%)	Vaginal dryness (17%)

(Continued)

Most common perimenopause symptoms (by percentage of women affected)	Most surprising perimenopause symptoms (by percentage of women affected)
Irritability (77%)	Mood swings (17%)
Low motivation (76%)	Acne or other skin issues (14%)
Joint pain (73%)	Tingling skin (14%)

Source: Women's Experiences of Perimenopause and Menopause (2024), Newson Health Research and Education

Instant expert

Kate Rowe-Ham on why doing nothing may cost you everything

Kate Rowe-Ham is a personal trainer, author, menopause coach and founder of Owning Your Menopause (owningyourmenopause.com).[12] *She helps women rebuild strength, confidence and identity in midlife, but believes men have a critical role to play in their transition and in recognizing their own.*

Many women want to walk away

There was a point where I wanted to pack my bags; I felt like I needed to go. Not because I didn't love him. But because I couldn't cope. It felt like I had spent years doing everything: the house, the kids, the cooking – the 'mental load' they call it – plus working. The reality is I never actually asked for help – almost like telepathically he should have known. Then the hormones hit. I changed. I cracked. But he didn't understand – why would he? Even I didn't, not really. I still looked like me. But that's what perimenopause does: it breaks you quietly, then quickly.

Small cracks become deep divides

It's not just about the cleaning. Or the laundry. Or the wet towels left on the floor. It's the weight of doing it all, every day, without acknowledgement. And when she's snaps, it's not about the dishwasher – it's about everything. It's a cry for help. But so many men miss the bigger picture.

Grow together – or grow apart

Your partner is changing – her body, her brain, her needs. If you're not evolving with her, you risk getting left behind. This isn't about being perfect. It's about being present, and a willingness to change, both individually and as a couple.

> **We both need a midlife reset**
>
> So many men tell me they feel flat, lost, or stuck, but they don't connect that to midlife. They think it's just stress or work or getting older. But it's hormonal. It's emotional. It's physical. And it's real. Men need to check in with themselves, too – not just to help her, but to fix their future.
>
> **You won't get a warning shot**
>
> So many men are blindsided when their partner walks away. But it doesn't come out of nowhere. Yes, we're good at hiding things. We can keep pushing on, even when we're falling apart. But if you really look, the signs are always there. The men that miss them just weren't paying any attention.

Piecing together the perimenopause puzzle

Knowing the symptoms is one thing. Spotting them in real life is another. They don't show up in an order. They don't tap you on the shoulder. They drift in and out – one lost train of thought at a time.

So it's time to channel your inner Poirot, Clouseau or Magnum PI – no moustache required.

Here's a breakdown of the perimenopause symptoms you're likely to notice first, grouped into common scenarios for faster recognition. These are the signs that start turning up in your house, your conversations and your relationship – often before she realizes what's going on.

1 The bedroom thermostat war

The sign: Hot flushes, night sweats and opening the windows to let in winter.

The scenario: You wake up freezing. She's drenched in sweat and leaning out the window, even though it's Narnia outside.

The science: Oestrogen helps regulate body temperature.[13] When levels drop, the body's internal thermostat becomes oversensitive, triggering sudden heat surges followed by chills. She's not exaggerating – her body thinks it's on fire.

Smoking Gun Score: ★★★★★

Classic sign. Hot flushes and night sweats are among the most recognizable early symptoms of oestrogen fluctuation – and perimenopause.

2 Mood swing city

The sign: Rage. Tears. Silence. Repeat.

The scenario: You're eating a packet of crisps. She looks at you like you just trod dog poo through the house.

The science: Oestrogen influences serotonin, dopamine and cortisol – the hormones that regulate mood, stress and impulse control.[14] When they spike or crash, emotions follow. Small things suddenly feel massive.

Smoking gun score: ★★★★☆
Strong possibility. It could also be stress, exhaustion or something else, but if it's new, intense and unpredictable, hormones are likely playing a big part (though couldn't you chew a little less loudly, mate?).

3 Lost for words

The sign: Brain fog, memory glitches, mid-sentence stalls.

The scenario: She's mid-story, mid-sentence and then … blank. Like someone just pulled the plug on her brain.

The science: Oestrogen supports cognitive function and memory processing.[15] When it declines, brain fog, forgetfulness and slower recall are common.

Smoking gun score: ★★★☆☆
Highly likely. That said, stress, poor sleep or overwork will scramble anyone's short-term memory. Look for a pattern, and what else is going on.

4 WTF warnings

The sign: Ringing ears, metallic taste, itchy skin, pins and needles – even changes to her sense of smell.

The scenario: Over dinner she told you her mouth tastes of blood, her foof is on fire, and your aftershave smells like a wet dog on a warm day. Happy anniversary.

The science: Hormonal changes can affect nerves, circulation and inflammation.[16] Some of her physical sensations may sound unbelievable to you, but they feel very real to her.

Smoking gun score: ★★★★☆
Very possible. A cluster of odd physical issues with no clear cause often points to hormonal shifts, but it's still worth checking with a GP to rule out anything else.

> **Itching to be understood**
>
> It's impossible for us to understand what a dry, itchy and sore vagina feels like, but let's try. Imagine wrapping your cock and balls with sandpaper, squeezing into a pair of denim shorts two sizes too small, then going about your business. All day. Every day. Now we're getting close.

5 The vanishing libido

The sign: Her sex drive's skipped town and left no forwarding address.

The scenario: OK, so you're more Wayne Rooney than George Clooney, but she used to rip your clothes off occasionally. Now when you make a move, she doesn't even roll over – she just stares at the ceiling like you suggested now's a good time to paint it.

The science: Testosterone and oestrogen affect desire, arousal and physical readiness for sex.[17] When they drop, libido often follows, and vaginal discomfort can make the thought of sex give her the ick. Chances are she'd genuinely prefer you to touch up that ceiling than her. But this isn't rejection – it's biology.

Smoking gun score: ★★★☆☆
Highly likely. Emotional stress, low mood or relationship tension can also affect libido – for her, as well as you (see Chapter 4) – but if other signs are showing up, too, hormones are the likely culprit.

6 Period chaos

The sign: Earlier. Later. Heavier. Longer. Mayhem.

The scenario: She hasn't said a word, but the hot water bottle looks exhausted and she's popping painkillers like they're Tic Tacs.

The science: Irregular periods are one of the most common signs of perimenopause.[18] Cycles can get shorter, longer, heavier or more intense. She might skip a period completely, then get hit with one that lasts two weeks and wipes her out. There's no pattern – just pandemonium.

Smoking gun score: ★★★★★
Almost certain. If her periods used to be regular but now aren't – especially alongside other symptoms – it's very likely perimenopause. But unless she brings it up, it's easy for you to miss. Stay tuned in.

7 She's become a stranger

The sign: She's flat, frightened or freaking out, and you never know which version will show up next.

The scenario: She used to hold everything – work, home, parents, kids, you – together without batting an eyelid. Now she's one burst bin bag away from a full-blown meltdown. And the worst part? She has no idea why life feels like it's spiralling out of control.

The science: This isn't just hormones messing with her emotions – they're messing with her sense of self. Oestrogen helps regulate stress, confidence and emotional resilience.[19] When it crashes, she might not recognize – or even like – the person she's becoming. And that's truly terrifying.

Smoking Gun Score: ★★★★☆
Very likely. If she's not herself – and she knows it – that's one of the clearest clues something's up. Your job? Don't panic. Stay steady. That's what she needs right now.

Same woman, new scent

If she suddenly smells different to you, you might not be imagining it.[20] Falling oestrogen can change her skin chemistry and sweat composition, so her bouquet might become stronger, sharper or even completely different. If she hasn't changed her deodorant or perfume, trust your nose – it might be onto something.

Real talk

'I'm a world champion athlete but had no idea what was happening to me'

I'm Christine. I'm 53, I live in Pennsylvania, and I'm a writer and founder of Wordshop, workshops in self-talk. I am also a Masters World Champion track cyclist and Peloton instructor and I've spent my life pushing limits – but nothing prepared me for menopause (christinedercole.com).

I thought the night sweats were just stress. They'd come and go since my thirties. I'd wake up drenched, confused, thinking, 'Did someone leave the oven on?' Then they'd vanish for six months and I'd think I was fine.

But around 51, it became undeniable. The sweats came nightly. The brain fog was relentless. I was misplacing things constantly – my wallet, my watch, even stuff I'd just had in my hand. I'd forget words mid-sentence. I'd create whole stories in my head about where things had gone, convinced I was losing my mind.

And the hardest part? I hadn't changed a thing. I was still training, still racing, still eating the same. But I gained weight, I hurt everywhere, and I didn't recognize my body – or myself. That was the most confusing thing. I've spent years telling women they are 'bigger than a smaller pair of pants' – and I believe that. But the truth? I still didn't want bigger pants. The emotional toll was real, and it caught me completely off guard. Recognizing that what was happening was indeed menopause was both heartbreaking and empowering. It's a process to reckon with the facts of ageing. And it is empowering to name a thing and be able to start a course of action to manage it.

Even once I started HRT, it didn't all click straight away. I'd lose the patches. When travelling, I would very consciously pack them in a specific spot, then could not remember what that spot was. It felt chaotic. But when I finally started talking about it during my Peloton classes, everything changed. I felt vulnerable speaking up, but when women messaged me saying, 'Thank you for saying it out loud', it was a real turning point. They felt seen. I felt seen.

This isn't the end of our usefulness. It's not the end of anything. But it can feel like it, especially if you're going through it alone. That's why I keep talking – so women feel seen. And men know how to stand beside them.

Reframing your reaction

You've started connecting the dots. Things are making more sense. But here's the next step – and it's a big one.

Because what you do with those clues – how you interpret and react to them – matters just as much as spotting them in the first place.

Up until now, how have you responded? Maybe not well. Even the most loving, loyal, switched-on partner can get it wrong, especially when her words or actions feel directed at you or catch you off guard.

But this isn't about blame – it's biology. And when you stop taking her behaviour at face value, and start seeing it through the lens of hormonal change, everything shifts. You can swap knee-jerk reactions for big-picture understanding and offer the support she needs. Let's break down the most common responses, what's really going on, and how to reframe your reaction. Because this is where connection deepens – or distance grows.

'She's overreacting'

Reframe it: *You're not under attack – her brain is.*
What looks like an overreaction is often her nervous system in overdrive. When oestrogen drops, the brain's ability to regulate emotion, stress and impulse control takes a hit.

Handle it: Don't meet fire with fire. Bring calm, not confrontation – it's the fastest way to bring her back down.

'She needs to calm down'

Reframe it: *That's not productive – it's provocation.*
Telling her to calm down when she's flooded with stress hormones is like pouring petrol on a barbecue. Her nervous system is already lit – don't fan the flames.

Handle it: Don't manage her emotions – manage the moment. Lower your voice, slow your breathing and really listen.

'She's just being moody'

Reframe it: *That's not a mood swing – it's a hormone whiplash.*
Hormones are pulling her mood in different directions, and it's impossible to maintain emotional balance.

Handle it: Treat it like the storm it is: stay calm and anchored, and wait until the worst of it passes.

'She loves drama'

Reframe it: *This isn't about attention – it's exhaustion.*
No woman volunteers for hot flushes, sleepless nights and panic attacks in the frozen food aisle. You couldn't fake it if you tried.

Handle it: Swap the cynicism for compassion. Take something off her plate, and stop treating her symptoms like a personality flaw.

'She's never up for anything anymore'

Reframe it: *She's not lazy – she's running on empty.*
Hormonal shifts drain energy, drive and motivation, and disrupt sleep and make recovery harder.

Handle it: She needs rest, not rejection. Protect her downtime so she can prioritize proper R&R.

'I can't do anything right'

Reframe it: *Don't take perimenopause personally.*
It might feel like you're always in the firing line, and maybe you are. But her frustration isn't about what you're getting right or wrong, it's about her feeling utterly out of control.

Handle it: Don't make it about you – we'll get to that in the next chapter. Right now, she needs stability, not sulking.

'She's gone cold on me'

Reframe it: *It's not rejection – it's withdrawal.*
She might not be pulling away from you; she's pulling away from everything. If she's lost her sense of self, that's a scary place to be.

Handle it: Don't huff. Don't puff. Show her she's loved without expecting sex, attention or anything in return. That's how to rebuild connection.

'She's not the woman I married'

Reframe it: *You're both changing – for the better.*
This isn't a glitch. It's growth. Her hormones are reshaping everything – her energy, her confidence, her needs, her boundaries. And the same goes for you (see Chapter 4).

Handle it: Stop looking for the woman she was; make space for one she's becoming. Ask her what she wants, and tell her what you need too. Understanding starts when you stop guessing.

'She's having an affair'

Reframe it: *Don't mistake distance for deception.*
Withdrawal, secrecy or lack of intimacy can feel suspicious, but they're often signs of fear, not infidelity. She may be shutting down because she doesn't have the words to explain how she's feeling.

Handle it: If she's pulling away, meet it with openness – not interrogation. Ask how she's feeling, not what she's hiding, and what she really needs from you now.

'She doesn't love me anymore'

Reframe it: *It's disconnection, not disappearance.*
Hormonal upheaval can flatten emotions, blunt desire, and leave her feeling numb, lonely or isolated, but that doesn't mean love is gone.

Handle it: Don't mirror the withdrawal. Stay kind, stay close, stay curious. This is the time for patience – not pressure.

Has her sex drive gone stratospheric?

The disappearance of libido is a very common complaint during perimenopause, but some women face the opposite 'problem': an unexpected surge in sexual desire that leaves exhausted partners begging for mercy before she starts burning through the vibrator batteries.

So what's behind her sudden case of *Stifler's Mom Syndrome*? As oestrogen levels rollercoaster during perimenopause, some women experience all-time hormonal highs – and that's when her sex drive can go into overdrive. It could also be the opposite: lower oestrogen levels mean testosterone has more influence, turning up the dial on mood and desire.

Still not convinced? Just check the dedicated Mumsnet threads, like we did.[21] But be warned – it's not for the faint-hearted. Here are just a few highlights:

> 'My poor husband is exhausted and begged me to just let him read his book last night.'

> 'I seem to suddenly like men who ooze testosterone – muscly, tall and bearded. Not my type normally.'
>
> 'Do I just go into another room and use a vibrator?! I had to wait for him to fall asleep. What is the etiquette for this sort of thing?'
>
> 'At one point I could barely stand to be near a handsome colleague who flirted with me. If you could die of lust, I'd be a corpse on the floor.'
>
> And these are just the tip of the, ahem, iceberg. You should read the ones we couldn't print – they're enough to make Madonna blush.

Why you matter more than you think

You've spotted the signs. You've reframed your reactions. That puts you in a unique position and makes you far more important than you think.

Because here's the uncomfortable truth: a lot of women still go through perimenopause alone and in silence. Their doctor shrugs. Their boss doesn't care. Their friends are dealing with their own chaos. That leaves their partner as the one person with the power to make a real difference. Yet most men either don't notice or don't know what to do. So they stay quiet, or bury their heads in the sand.

Lucky for her, you're not 'most men'.

Before you break the ice ...

You've paid attention. You've joined the dots. You've stepped up when it would've been far easier to step back. Your role now isn't to be perfect, but it is to be purposeful.

In the next section, we'll show you how to break the ice and have conversations that bring you closer together – and help you handle whatever life throws your way.

But there's one thing we need to talk about first: you.

Because let's be honest – this isn't just her storm. You're in it, too. And whether you're steadying the ship or screaming at the sky could be the difference between making it to calmer waters or going under together.

... Take a look in the mirror

That's right – this is all just as much about you as it is her.

We know that might sound strange right now. You've been focused on spotting her symptoms, making sense of her changes, and trying to offer some tentative support. But here's the thing: a lot of what she's feeling? You might be feeling too. The fatigue. The low mood. The brain fog. The dip in sex drive. The nagging sense that something's changed, but you can't quite put your finger on what.

Sound familiar? You're not going crazy. Midlife hits hard – for both of you. And while her symptoms might be centre stage in your thoughts, yours won't stay in the wings for ever.

So now we need to take a moment to check in with you. And that makes the next chapter arguably the most important in the whole book. Why? Because the best way to show up for her? Start showing up for yourself first.

4

OK, but what about me?
Men, mojo and the midlife crisis

You've seen what's happening to her – but what about you? Midlife has a way of pulling the rug without warning. Your body's changing, your brain's buffering, and the old tricks for feeling good don't work like they used to. No one told you this was coming – and be honest, when was the last time anyone asked you how you're really doing?

This chapter takes a microscope to what's really going on with you – the hormonal changes, the identity crisis, the creeping sense of drift – and reveals how you can rebuild yourself stronger. Not to be the man you once were but to become the one you've always wanted to be.

In this chapter you'll discover:

- What low testosterone actually feels like and when to get it tested
- Whether the male menopause – or 'manopause' – really exists
- How to tell the difference between a hormonal dip and a midlife crisis
- Why libido goes missing in midlife and how to get yours back
- How to find your life's 'second mountain' and why it's worth the climb
- How sorting yourself is the first step to supporting her better
- Why a midlife wobbly might just be the turning point you've been waiting for.

By now, you've seen what she's dealing with – the brain fog, low mood, poor sleep, anxiety, irritability, stubborn weight gain, vanishing libido and that unnerving sense of disconnection. But here's the thing: how many of those feel familiar?

Be honest: are you feeling them, too? Tired all the time. Snapping at things that used to wash over you. Going through the motions. No energy. No spark. No hard-on. No idea of what you're doing, what you want, or where it all went wrong.

This chapter is about that. It's about you. About the physical changes that creep up without warning: the slow drop in testosterone, the rising stress, the belly fat that won't shift, the fog that doesn't lift. But it's also about something deeper. The midlife drift. The loss of purpose. The constant worry over why you don't feel like yourself anymore.

You're not broken. You're not weak. You're not alone. But you are in transition. Just like her. And you deserve a little TLC, too. This chapter unpacks what's happening to your hormones, your identity and your sense of direction, so you can make sense of the chaos and find your way back to resilience, drive and connection – and put the glory back in your mornings.

What's the story?

The good news? You're not going mad. You're just in midlife.

The bad news? No one warns you it's coming or how strange it feels. Especially when you were banking on becoming a sophisticated silver fox, not a balding grizzly bear with a bad back and a beer belly.

Suddenly, you're tired all the time. Snapping at things that never used to bother you. You can't sleep, can't focus and can't be arsed – avoiding the stuff you used to enjoy: sex, sport, spontaneity. Your brain's like a browser with 47 open tabs – and none is responding. And every part of you aches all the time, even though your gym membership lapsed back when people thought an air fryer was a type of jet engine, not the fastest way to cook sausages.

You feel foggy, flat, flabby and you've misplaced your mojo. Something's shifted. You just don't know what. But you're not the only one who feels a little bit … lost.

> ### Real talk
>
> **'I lost who I was – but found who I needed to be'**
>
> *I'm Mike. I'm 45, I live in Leeds, and I'm the co-founder of Unify (unify-men.com), a men's coaching platform helping guys navigate the challenges of midlife with clarity, purpose and connection (mikebates.uk).*
>
> I'd spent 20 years leading within elite military and Ministry of Defence covert operations. High stakes. High standards. High purpose. I was clear on who I was, what I did, and why it mattered. Then one day, it was over – and I had no idea what came next.
>
> I didn't realize it at the time, but I was grieving. Not for people – for purpose. I didn't know who I was without the uniform, the team, the mission. I wasn't depressed in the clinical sense. Just flat. Disconnected. Directionless. I couldn't find my place in the world, and I didn't know how to ask for help.
>
> The hardest part? From the outside, everything looked fine. But inside, I was drifting. I'd built my identity around performance, protection, pushing through. Suddenly none of that applied and I had no roadmap. No role. No idea how to start again.
>
> I had to rebuild from the ground up. Let go of who I'd been and figure out who I actually wanted to be. Not just for me but for the people around me.
>
> That's what led me to start Unify. I didn't want other men to go through what I did in silence. Midlife isn't a crisis – it's a chance to get honest, reconnect, and build something real and lasting. But that opportunity only happens once you have the courage to stop pretending you've got it all handled.

When hormones and habits collide

So what's going on? Your hormones might be part of the problem. So might your habits.[1] So might the creeping dread that this – work, doomscroll, sleep, repeat – is all there is.

The fix? It starts with figuring out what's really going on. And sometimes, it's simpler than you think. Strength training, for example, isn't just good for your body – it's a proven way to reboot your hormones,[2] rebuild your identity,[3] and rewire your brain for greater resilience (see Chapter 11).[4] So, you don't need a new life. You just need a new approach.

> ### Testosterone 101
>
> #### What it does, what can go wrong – and how to fix it
>
> Testosterone has a bad-boy reputation as the hormone behind beards, brawling and bonking, but the reality is more complex. Yes, it's the key driver of male physical development – making us bigger, stronger, faster and hairier than women.[5] But it also plays a central role in energy, focus, mood, motivation, confidence, fat distribution, metabolism, sleep and more.[6] When testosterone is low, you don't just feel less like a man – you feel less like yourself. Here's what you need to know.
>
> **What is testosterone?** It's the primary male sex hormone.[7] Produced mainly in the testicles, it's regulated by a hormonal loop involving your brain, specifically the hypothalamus and pituitary gland. Most of the testosterone in your body is bound to proteins like SHBG (sex hormone-binding globulin), making it inactive.[8] Only a small fraction circulates as 'free testosterone', and that's what drives how you feel and function day to day.
>
> **What does testosterone do?** Testosterone helps build muscle, burn fat, sharpen focus, regulate mood, boost motivation, and maintain energy, sleep quality and emotional resilience. When levels fall, everything can take a hit, especially how you perform in the weights room, the meeting room and the bedroom.[9]
>
> **Why do I need it?** Without enough, your physical, mental and emotional wellbeing starts to unravel. Low testosterone can leave you tired, foggy, flabby, demotivated and disconnected – not just from sex, but from your sense of self.[10]
>
> **When does it peak – and why does it decline?** Testosterone peaks in your late teens to early twenties, when your body is primed for growth, drive and reproduction. From your thirties onwards, it starts to decline gradually – around 1–2 percent a year.[11] That drop-off accelerates with poor sleep, high stress, excess fat and inactivity. Symptoms often show up in your forties or fifties, especially if a sedentary and stressful lifestyle has taken its toll.[12]

What are the warning signs of low T? Your sex drive drops.[13] You feel tired, foggy and flat. You gain belly fat, lose muscle, struggle with sleep, and snap more easily than usual. You might feel like a duller, quieter version of yourself – less focused, less motivated, and less connected to the people or things that used to matter. More than one in three men over 45 have clinically low testosterone levels, according to large-scale studies.[14]

Can I fix it naturally? For most men, yes. Regular strength training, better sleep, reducing stress, improving your diet, losing excess fat and cutting alcohol can all help bring testosterone levels back into a healthy range – especially if you're borderline low.[15] Healthier habits can also make any future testosterone replacement treatment (TRT) more effective.[16]

What if that's not enough? If your symptoms persist and blood tests show a genuine testosterone deficiency, TRT may help[17] – and it can be life-changing.[18] But there are considerations – TRT requires proper medical supervision, regular monitoring and a long-term commitment. And it's not cheap – you'll probably have to cough up yourself because the NHS and many private healthcare plans won't cover it.[19]

When hormones wreak havoc

So, testosterone is starting to decline – slowly at first, then faster if you're stressed, knackered, or your paunch has got its own postcode.

Cortisol – the main stress hormone – is on the rise.[20] That means disrupted sleep, shorter patience, and a constant simmering rage usually reserved for people who think the whole train carriage wants to hear their Spotify playlist.

Insulin resistance might be creeping up, too, leading to more belly fat, more cravings, more fatigue, and less control over your energy, mood and motivation.[21]

And all of this is happening at once. You're physically, mentally and emotionally drained. This isn't only about hormones, but it's not just in your head either.

It sounds a lot like perimenopause, except it's happening to you. Some people call it the 'manopause', but is that a thing? And if not, what the hell is going on?

> ### Andropause 101
>
> **Is the 'manopause' real?**
>
> It's been called the manopause, andropause and even the male menopause. But here's the truth: it's not the same – not even close.[22]
>
> Most experts dislike the comparison – and the implication.[23] It suggests a dramatic hormonal event on par with menopause, when in reality the decline is slow, inconsistent and not experienced by every man. It also risks trivializing the very real, often life-changing symptoms many women face during their far more extreme biological events.
>
> The real issue? Many men experience symptoms – brain fog, fatigue, low mood, poor sleep, belly fat, irritability, low libido, and a drop in drive, resilience and connection – without understanding the cause. And because testosterone testing[24] and treatment[25] are still poorly handled by many doctors,[26] they're often left misdiagnosed, medicated for the wrong problem, or simply told to 'man up'. To make matters worse, some of the most common and obvious symptoms of low testosterone – poor sleep,[27] high stress,[28] weight gain[29] – can also drive levels down further, creating a vicious feedback loop that goes unnoticed, untested and untreated. If you feel off and nothing adds up, don't ignore it.

There's no 'manopause', but the feel is real

It's tempting to call it the male menopause – if we give it a name, maybe it has a straightforward solution. Now it's not just about what's gone 'wrong' with you.

The reality? Men don't go through the same hormonal horror show as women. What you're experiencing is real, but it's not menopause. It's something slower and more subtle, and hormones alone can't carry the can. But there is a way out, and it starts by climbing the metaphorical mountain standing between you and a healthier, happier second half of your life.

Sex drive, libido, the horn: Has your desire done a runner?

When your sex drive disappears, it's easy to panic or pretend nothing's wrong. But libido is often the first red flag that your hormones, health or headspace are out of sync. Because, despite what you might think – or, erm, feel – sexual desire starts in your brain, not in your boxer shorts.

Hormones play a big part. Testosterone drives libido in both men and women – not just by increasing physical arousal but by influencing motivation, confidence, and reward-seeking behaviour.[30] If T drops, so does drive.

So while desire can be dulled by low testosterone, the real damage often comes from stress, belly fat, poor sleep and the slow erosion of confidence or connection.[31] If you're constantly anxious, wired or knackered, your brain's going to prioritize survival, not sexy time.[32]

In women, oestrogen helps keep vaginal tissue healthy, and supports mood and emotional connection, which are critical to desire. When her oestrogen and testosterone crash – alongside exhaustion, resentment or communication breakdown – libido can take a nosedive,[33] especially if sex has become painful[34] or uncomfortable or just feels like another job on her never-ending to-do list.

No spark, no shame – but don't ignore it

There's no 'normal' sex drive, and no magic number of times you should be in the mood.[35] But if desire has vanished for six months or more, or you feel disconnected from intimacy, you should find out why.[36] That's the point at which doctors recommend seeking help – especially if the loss of interest is causing distress or affecting your relationship.

Bottom line? Hormones don't work alone. They're shaped by sleep, stress, mood, body image – and whatever's happening (or not happening) in your relationship. If your sex drive has gone AWOL, start there. Fix the foundations (see Chapter 9) and it may come roaring back. Low libido isn't failure: it's feedback. So tune in – don't zone out.

Is it hormones – or something deeper?

It's common for men to feel lost in midlife,[37] and it's easy to blame low testosterone. Sometimes it is the reason. But hormones don't explain everything. Because this stage of life doesn't just mess with your biology – it messes with your identity. Your role, your purpose, your place in the world. That quiet voice in your head asking, 'Is this really it?' gets louder.

You might be low on testosterone. You might be stuck in a midlife rut. It might be both. But if you want to take back control, you need to stop guessing and start getting answers.

Low T or midlife crisis?

Low testosterone is a biological issue with a measurable cause. It's rooted in hormones, not habits, and needs medical evaluation. The symptoms, as we've covered, can be physical (muscle loss, low libido, weaker erections), mental (brain fog, low mood, disconnection), or both.

A midlife crisis isn't hormonal – it's existential.[38] It's what happens when purpose fades, routine take over, and life feels smaller than it should. It's something you fix with ongoing introspection, not weekly injections.

In short, one's in your blood. The other's in your soul. Knowing the difference is how you start to turn things around. Here's how to tell them apart, despite the overlaps:

Low T	Midlife malaise
Zero sex drive	Feeling stuck or like you're going nowhere
Weak, unreliable, or no erections	You've lost your sense of purpose or identity
Belly fat won't shift, muscles fading	You feel invisible – at work, at home, in life
Exhausted, even after a full night's sleep	You numb out with booze, scrolling or overwork
Brain fog, can't focus	You feel emotionally disconnected, even from your partner
Flat, joyless, emotionally shut down	You've stopped caring about the things you used to
Poor recovery from workouts	You keep thinking, 'What's the point?'
No motivation, no drive, no spark	Bored, restless, doubting everything

Midlife crisis 101

Down and out in the valley of doubt

Forget the clichés about getting a Ferrari, squeezing into skinny jeans and running off with your secretary. A midlife crisis isn't about vanity – it's about identity. Specifically, the slow, silent disappearance of the man you thought you were. You built a life. A career. An identity. You wore it like armour. Now it doesn't fit ... and underneath? There's nothing.

You climbed the first mountain, and no one told you there'd be a second one. It's an idea popularized by David Brooks in his book *The Second Mountain: The quest for a moral life* – a shift from ego and achievement to purpose and contribution.[39] Less chasing status, more helping others rise. If that appeals to you, keep reading.

Free-falling into the abyss

The first half of your life is the first mountain. That's where you chase all the things young men are taught to value: power, status, success and respect.[40] You work hard, climb fast, live in the moment. You build your career, win promotions, earn money, raise kids, buy a house. The rules are simple – life is a competition: do more, earn more, achieve more.

Then one day, you hit the top. You've done everything you were told would make you happy. The boxes are all ticked – career, house, kids, income. Instead of feeling triumphant, you feel ... nothing. It doesn't feel like success. It feels like emptiness. And before you realize it, you've passed the peak and started sliding down the other side. There's no new challenge, no higher summit – just a slow, quiet descent into frustration, fatigue and the stomach-churning fear that this isn't how your life was meant to be. Welcome to the midlife crisis canyon.

Life in the valley can look like apathy, withdrawal or restlessness – and feel like overwhelm, detachment or a nagging sense that something's not right. Left unchecked, it slowly erodes your motivation, strains your relationships, and drains the joy from your life.

Summit the second mountain

And then, just when you think you've hit rock bottom, you realize something: there's another mountain. A second one. And the only way forward is up.

This time, the climb is different. You're no longer chasing power, money or approval. You're building something deeper – a life shaped by purpose, connection and meaning.

It's not about what you can prove. It's about what you can pass on – your time, your wisdom, your presence – to help others rise. That's the second mountain. And the view as you climb? It's worth every step.

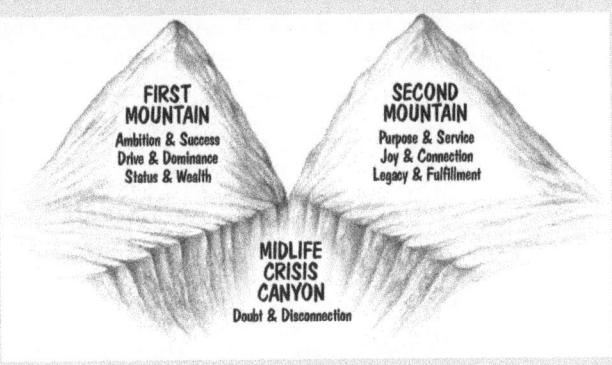

From breakdown to breakthrough

Now you know what a midlife crisis really is – not a cliché, but a changing of identity – it's time to take action. If you're convinced it's all down to testosterone, hold that thought – we'll get to the blood tests and treatment options soon. But first, let's get your head and heart back on track.

> **Instant expert**
>
> ### Mike Bates on how to overcome a midlife crisis
>
> *Mike Bates, who we first met earlier in this chapter, knows what it means to lose your identity – and build it back better. After a 20-year career, the former covert counter-terrorism operations leader within the intelligence and security fields of the UK's Ministry of Defence co-founded Unify (unifymen.com) to help men face the midlife minefield head-on – and come out the other side with clarity, courage and connection (mikebates.uk).*
>
> **Identity loss is common – but not forever**
>
> Most men hit a point in midlife where they no longer recognize the person in the mirror. The identity that served them in the first half of life –

the role of provider, protector, career man – suddenly doesn't fit. They feel flat, directionless or invisible, but can't explain why. This is normal. You're not broken. You've simply outgrown the identity that used to define you. And that presents an opportunity: now is the time to figure out who you really are and who you want to be next.

Midlife isn't a crisis – it's a transition

The so-called midlife crisis is really a crossroads – the moment you realize the life you've built isn't giving you what it used to. That's not failure. It's feedback. You've climbed the first mountain – career, status, family – and now you're standing at the foot of the second, asking yourself what matters to you now. The men who thrive in the second half of life are the ones who stop trying to relive the past and start writing a new story.

You can't buy your way out of feeling lost

When men lose their sense of self, they often reach for distractions – cars, clothes, watches. But you can't spend your way out of an identity crisis. The real work is internal. What matters now isn't how you look or what you earn – it's who you are when no one's watching. Midlife can feel like a void, but it's also an invitation – to stop chasing things you thought you needed and start building the life you actually want.

Shame loves silence – so start talking

Feeling stuck, useless or irrelevant isn't a shortcoming – it's being human. But most men don't talk about it because we've been conditioned to stay silent. That silence breeds shame, and shame keeps you isolated. The greatest courage any man can have is to be vulnerable – to be honest about what's really going on behind the mask. That's not a weakness. That's real strength – far greater than bravado, control or keeping it all in.

You hold the pen – so you write your future

It doesn't matter how successful you've been, or how far off track you've drifted. You get to choose what the second half of your life looks like. That choice might feel impossible when you're exhausted or burnt out, but it starts with small actions, not grand gestures. Better health. Better sleep. Better conversations. The next 45 years can be the best yet – not despite what you've been through, but because of it. You just have to decide to show up.

Scaling the second mountain: Your quick-start guide

You don't need to quit your job, sell everything you own, and go and live off-grid in a yurt. But you do need to get back to basics. Because finding your second-mountain motivation isn't about reinvention – it's about remembering who you really are beneath the weight of your daily routines and responsibilities. Here's where to start – and remember: the second mountain isn't climbed in a day, but every choice takes you further from the valley below. This isn't the end of the story – it's the start of your defining chapter.

1 **Audit your energy.** What gives you energy? What drains it? Start by doing more of the first and less of the second.
2 **Reconnect with meaning.** What did you care about before life got noisy or numb? Creativity? Coaching? Adventure? People? Your purpose is probably hiding in your past.
3 **Have the conversation.** Tell someone how you're feeling – warts and all. Not a WhatsApp message or a rushed pint. A proper, honest conversation with a close mate, a coach or a therapist.
4 **Set a 'second mountain' goal.** The rules: choose something that scares you a little. That requires growth, not ego. That benefits others, not just yourself.
5 **Don't wait to feel ready.** If you do, you'll be waiting for ever. Take small steps. Try new things. Keep showing up. Clarity will follow.

> **Who you gonna call?**
>
> Life got you by the balls and you don't know who to talk to? Picture this: you've been taken hostage by a gang of heavily armed drug smugglers deep in the Amazon rainforest. They're – somehow – immune to your charm, wit and encyclopaedic knowledge of *The Sopranos*. You get one phone call to save your skin. Who do you ring? That's your guy.

The truth about testosterone

You've taken the time to reconnect with your values, passions and purpose but you still feel off? Then chances are it's not your life that's off track – it's your hormones. The only way to know for sure is to get it tested. Don't worry – we'll explain everything you need to know. But first, let's explore what low testosterone actually is and why problems with testing mean many men don't get the help they need.

What is low T?

Understanding your blood test results is the first step to making sense of your options, but before you start analysing your numbers, you need to know that testosterone is measured differently depending on where you live. The UK and most of the rest of the world reports testosterone levels in nanomoles per litre (nmol/L),[41] but the US uses nanograms per decilitre (ng/dL).[42]

What your T count really means

Confused by your results? Here's how to decode them, and what each range says about your symptoms, treatment options and next steps.[43]

Testosterone	UK & rest of world (nmol/L)	US	What it means
Very Low	Below 8	Below 230	Symptoms likely. Medical review strongly advised. Often qualifies for NHS TRT.
Low / Borderline	8–12	230–350	May cause symptoms. Often denied NHS treatment. Common qualifying range privately.
Normal / Average	13–30	351–870	Considered healthy range. TRT unlikely to be offered unless symptoms are severe.
High	Over 30	Over 870	Can occur naturally or through over-supplementation. Monitor for health risks.

Note: Testosterone levels can vary by lab, testing method and time of day. These ranges are general guidelines only. Diagnosis and treatment should always be guided by a qualified healthcare professional.

> Instant expert

Dr Jeff Foster on the truth about testosterone testing

Dr Jeff Foster is an NHS GP and Director of Men's Health at online health testing and treatment platform Voy/Manual. He's spent his career calling out the confusion, clichés and wrong calls around male hormones and helping men get the answers and support they actually need (drjefffoster.co.uk).

Don't wait until it's too late

Most men don't come and see me until they're on their knees. They're burnt out. Depressed. Their relationship's broken down. They feel lost. And all the while, they think they just have to push through. But once they get a proper workup – a full set of blood tests and a detailed health review – it can be transformative. They feel like themselves again.

Most GPs don't test properly

On the NHS, at best, you'll usually get a total testosterone test. Often, it's taken at the wrong time of day, when levels are lower. That's no good. If you are under 40, testosterone should be tested in the early morning. And total T isn't enough in many cases. You may also need free T, sex hormone-binding globulin (SHBG), luteinizing hormone (LH) and follicle-stimulating hormone (FSH) – alongside other key markers like prolactin, thyroid function and HbA1c (a measure of long-term blood sugar control and insulin resistance). Without these, it's not a full assessment, and you may be told everything is normal, when, in fact, your available testosterone is low.

Prepare to go private

If you've been feeling off for weeks and there's no obvious cause like grief, burnout or a new baby, stop trying to power through. Get tested. A proper blood test can give you answers you won't get from willpower alone. Just be warned: if you want a full picture, you may need to go private. That means spending money, but it also means ending the cycle of guesswork, frustration, and feeling like a shadow of your former self.

A normal result isn't the all-clear

Blood tests can come back in the normal range but you still feel awful. That range is huge, and symptoms matter more than scores. Good hormone care doesn't start with TRT. It starts with a proper look at your weight, sleep, diet, stress and alcohol intake. Testosterone replacement is never the first move. It's the last resort – once everything else has been ruled out or addressed.

It's not just how you feel – it's your future health

T isn't just about libido or energy. Chronically low levels are linked to insulin resistance, increased fat mass, type-2 diabetes, reduced bone strength, and a higher risk of cardiovascular disease. It also affects mental health and emotional regulation – which can trigger depression, anxiety and relationship breakdowns. The symptoms might feel bearable now, but the long-term impact is real. Don't brush it off. You're not just fixing your libido – you're reclaiming the rest of your life.

What is TRT – and do you need it?

TRT is booming – and it's not just gym bros and porn stars chasing a boost. In 2023 almost $2 billion (£1.5 billion) was spent on testosterone treatments in the US alone – a figure expected to rise to $3 billion by 2033.[44]

As awareness grows, stigma fades, and more men get tested, there's a growing recognition that low T is a diagnosable and treatable problem.

Yet it remains misunderstood by many. Yes, it can be life-changing – for the right man, at the right dose, under the right guidance.[45] But it's not a magic bullet, nor a short-term fix, and it's not right for everyone.[46]

If you suspect you have low T, or have the blood results to prove it, here are the answers to the most common TRT questions to help you decide whether it's the right move for you.

What does TRT do?

TRT is a treatment to restore testosterone levels if yours have dropped below a healthy range and are causing symptoms. It's not about boosting you to superhuman status – it's about getting you back to where you should be.

Do I qualify for TRT?

On the NHS, you'll usually only qualify if your total testosterone is below 8 nmol/L (nanomoles per litre) on at least two separate morning blood tests, and you're showing clear symptoms.[47] Even then, getting treatment can be tricky:[48] many GPs are reluctant to prescribe TRT because of limited training, outdated concerns about safety, or the commitment of prescribing a lifelong medication. Most men with borderline or moderately low levels will need to go private, where the threshold to qualify for treatment can be double that of the NHS (see below).

> ### CV or eulogy: How do you want to be remembered?
> What if your gradual decline in testosterone isn't an ending but a recalibration? A slow hormonal shift that allows you to become something more: a man who leads not through intimidation but with wisdom. From Carl Jung's *Senex*,[49] Lars Tornstam's *Gerotranscendence* theory,[50] and David Brooks' *Second Mountain* (see above), the 'Wise Elder' is a familiar role in psychology and culture, inviting men of a certain age to trade ego and ambition for introspection, restraint, perspective, purpose and legacy.
>
> In short, Brooks asks: How do you want to be remembered? By the lines on your CV – or by the lives you've touched?
>
> Maybe a drop in T – as long as it's not clinically low – isn't the problem it's made out to be. Maybe it's the unexpected invitation you've been waiting for.

How does TRT work?

TRT adds testosterone to your body to replace what it's no longer making in sufficient amounts.[51] This can ease symptoms like fatigue, brain fog, low libido and poor recovery, but only if your levels are genuinely low and you've already addressed any lifestyle issues that could be dragging you down.

How long does TRT take to work?

Some men notice a lift in energy, mood or sex drive within a few weeks.[52] For others, it takes longer. Most will need to wait 3–6 months to feel the full benefits. TRT isn't a quick fix – it's a slow and steady recalibration.

How do I take TRT?

There are a few options, but there's no one-size-fits-all.[53] Your dosage, delivery method and frequency need to be tailored to you and monitored by a specialist. Typical options are:

- gels or creams applied daily to the skin
- injections every 2–12 weeks, or microdoses several times a week
- patches, changed daily
- pellet implants (inserted under the skin in the buttocks or hips), lasting 3–6 months, although these are less common.

How much does TRT cost?

If you can't access TRT through the NHS or private health insurance, you'll have to pay – and it's not cheap. In the UK, gels, creams or injections typically cost £80–£150 per month.[54] Pellet implants cost £400–£800 per insertion, but last many months. Add-on costs include blood tests (£50–£150 each) and fertility-preserving drugs, like HCG (£30–£40 per month).

In the US, it's often more expensive. Monthly treatment plans range from $100 to $500, with blood tests usually $100 or more.[55]

Is TRT safe?

It's not suitable for men with active prostate or breast cancer,[56] and certain other health conditions may also rule it too.[57] Otherwise, yes – if it's prescribed and properly monitored. Side effects can include acne, irritability and disturbed sleep, especially at first,[58] along with shrinking testicles over time. TRT reduces sperm production, so you may need extra medication if you're trying for a baby. And because it suppresses your body's own testosterone, TRT is a long-term commitment. Once you're on it, you'll likely need it for life.

Wait – my balls will shrink?

They might. TRT can shrink your testicles because it shuts down your body's own testosterone production, but it's usually harmless.[59] If preserving fertility or natural testosterone is important to you, talk to your doctor about extra meds like HCG or enclomiphene to keep everything downstairs in good working order.

Can you get TRT for free?

Because the NHS only approves TRT for men with very low testosterone, if you're on the border you might miss out, even if your symptoms are severe. Private clinics have far more relaxed thresholds, and you may find some private providers flag results as 'low' even though NHS guidelines say you're fine. They often also place more weight on symptoms than scores[60] – a cynic might claim that's because they have a clear financial incentive to treat as many men as possible. Ultimately, you're far more likely to get TRT if you're willing to pay for it.

Is TRT the solution you need?

TRT can help – sometimes dramatically. But as you now know, it's never the first step. And it's not for everyone. That's why rushing straight to treatment without a full picture is risky.

Because here's the truth: plenty of men with textbook testosterone levels still feel awful, yet others with low readings feel fine.[61] That's why real diagnosis is about more than numbers – it's about symptoms, context, and the stuff blood tests can't tell you.

Instant expert

Dr Ben Davis on how to know if you really need TRT

Dr Ben Davis is a straight-talking GP and sex and relationship therapist expert who helps men separate real symptoms from midlife marketing scams and take back control of their health and happiness (drben.uk).

Low T isn't always a problem

Testosterone does decline with age, but your levels are affected by everything from genetics to fat mass to sleep quality. It doesn't always cause symptoms – that's why proper diagnosis is based on symptoms, not just a number on a lab test. Don't get obsessed with blood tests – pay attention to how you feel.

TRT helps – but only if it's the right tool

TRT can be transformative for men with symptomatic low T. But it won't fix a life that's out of sync. If you're under-slept, unfit, overweight and overstressed, TRT won't cover the cracks. The lifestyle foundations must come first – quality sleep, regular exercise, a decent diet, dedicated downtime and social connection. If not, TRT is just a very expensive cream. Fix the habits first, then test, then treat – if it's really needed.

Body fat lowers T – more than getting older

One of the biggest drivers of low testosterone isn't time – it's circumference. Excess body fat, especially around the belly, leads to higher oestrogen and lower testosterone. And the most effective way to reverse it? Strength training. Lifting weights boosts natural testosterone production, reduces body fat, improves sleep, lowers stress, and gives you structure, focus and purpose. So, if you want higher T levels, start getting strong.

Get tested – but don't get hustled

Most men with borderline levels won't qualify for TRT on the NHS – unless they have very low readings or a diagnosed issue like testicular failure. That's where private clinics come in and where things get murky. Many use social media and slick sales tactics to market fear, then push TRT as an easy fix for fatigue and low mood to sell you an ongoing subscription package. TRT is for life – so, if you stop, your symptoms return. Always listen to good medical advice, not a 30-second sales pitch.

TRT trap: How to spot a shady clinic

Testosterone treatment is big business, so it's no wonder so many new providers are popping up to try to cash in on the craze. While there are many brilliant online clinics staffed by passionate, patient-focused doctors, some are more motivated by maximizing profits than delivering life-changing care. Here are the red flags to watch out for so you don't end up wasting your money or harming your health.

- **They don't ask about your symptoms.** If they jump straight to prescribing based on a single blood test result, without asking how you feel, watch out. A good clinic looks at the whole picture – not just your numbers.

- **They don't do a full blood test.** Some clinics only check total testosterone, which isn't enough. To properly assess hormone health, you need a full panel: sex hormone-binding globulin, luteinizing hormone, follicle-stimulating hormone, prolactin, thyroid function and HbA1c. And, for accuracy, your blood test should be done between 7 AM and 11 AM, and repeated at least once, ideally a week apart.[62]
- **They skip over lifestyle fixes.** A good expert will tell you poor sleep, stress, obesity and booze often cause low T. If they don't mention fixing those before starting treatment, they're only interested in your cash.
- **They sell TRT as a miracle cure.** TRT is a long-term solution – not a quick fix. If the marketing promises instant energy, incredible sex and six-pack abs and doesn't mention it's a lifelong commitment, they're selling fantasy, not pharmaceuticals.
- **They don't mention side effects or risks.** Shrinking testicles, suppressed fertility, acne, mood swings – these need to be discussed up front. If they're not transparent or balanced, walk away.
- **They don't offer regular monitoring.** TRT needs ongoing blood tests and medical oversight. If there's no clear follow-up plan, they don't care about your long-term health.
- **They push expensive extras you don't understand.** Steer clear of clinics trying to upsell stacks of pricey supplements, peptides or other 'biohacks' without explaining what they do or why you might need them.
- **They rely on influencers or clickbait sales funnels.** Best-practice healthcare isn't sold on TikTok reels or Instagram posts. If it feels more like a marketing campaign than a medical service, trust your gut.
- **You never speak to the same doctor twice.** Continuity of care matters for ongoing treatment. If you're bounced between different clinicians, it's hard to get proper care.

You've both changed – now what?

So, you've figured out what's going on. You've identified the issues and taken the first steps towards feeling like yourself again. Stronger. Sharper. More in control.

And somewhere along the way, you've probably started connecting the dots. The things you've been feeling – the fatigue, the brain fog, the short fuse, the low libido, the restless 'What's it all for?' feeling – aren't all that different from what she's been going through. In fact, they're almost exactly the same.

Midlife doesn't discriminate. It hits your hormones, your identity, your confidence and your connection, and it tends to hit both of you at once. She's burning up. You're frozen out. Same storm, different ships.

The reality is that you've both changed. She might not feel like the woman you married, but you might not be the man she first met either. There's no blame. It's biology and life catching up with you.

When that penny drops, it can be overwhelming. Fixing one of you felt hard enough – but both of you? At the same time? No wonder divorce rates for couples in their fifties are soaring.[63]

Support starts with you

There's a light at the end of the tunnel – and it's not an oncoming train. There might even be something strangely reassuring in realizing you're not in this alone. Right now, you might be the target of each other's rage, fears and frustrations. And you probably can't remember the last time you held hands – let alone anything more intimate.

But this isn't the end. It's a turning point.

Because here's what really matters: you can't support her if you're falling apart too. Understanding what's going on in your own mind and body isn't selfish – it's essential. When you're steadier, stronger and more self-aware, you're far better placed to show up for her in the ways she needs most.

And it's not about choosing between her needs and yours – it's about recognizing that both matter. The more you understand about what's really happening – to you and to her – the easier it becomes to talk honestly, navigate the chaos, and figure out what you both need to make it through.

In the next chapter, we'll show you how to ride out the emotional rollercoaster without wrecking the relationship. You'll learn what to do when the mood swings, meltdowns or misunderstandings come out of nowhere – and how to stay calm when she can't.

And after that? We begin rebuilding – with the kind of communication that doesn't just patch things up but helps you reconnect, reset, and face the future on the same team.

Part 2
COMMUNICATION

5

Riding the emotional rollercoaster
Keeping your cool when everything's up in the air

You've seen how midlife and menopause can rattle both of you – physically, emotionally and relationally. Now comes the biggest challenge: holding it together when everything feels like it's falling apart. This chapter is your guide to staying steady when things start to spiral. It's about keeping your head when she's losing hers. Extinguishing the flames, not fanning them. Staying grounded, not walking on eggshells. Because before you can fix what's gone wrong, you have to survive the fallout. Only then can you start the conversations that change everything.

In this chapter you'll discover:

- How to handle the heat without losing your cool
- What she really means when she says 'All you care about is yourself' or 'I feel so ugly'
- The five flashpoint phrases most likely to spark a row – and how to defuse them fast
- The 12 science-backed hacks to stay calm when you're about to blow
- Why keeping quiet sometimes matters more than being right
- How to step back without looking like you're checking out.

We owe you an apology. The first section of this book wasn't exactly a barrel of laughs, was it?

We've covered brain freezes, red-hot fury, sex drive slumps, and sleep that's rarer than hen's teeth – not to mention your stuff: the apathy, the restlessness, the questioning of who you really are, and what the hell you're going to do with the rest of your life.

It's a lot.

And while we've explained why it's all happening, we haven't said what you can do about it. Nothing. Nada. Zilch. Zip. Don't worry – that changes in the next chapter. From then on, we're all about giving you the tools, strategies and confidence to turn things around. Promise.

Survive first, then solve

But before we hand you the keys to the happier life you want, there's one thing you need to know: nothing's going to get better if you don't survive the current carnage.

The reality is that for most midlife couples, half the battle is simply staying together long enough to reach the point where you're both ready, willing and able to properly talk about what's really going on – rather than only ever communicating through stunned silence, slammed doors or an expensive lawyer.

If we had to summarize the point of this chapter in two words, it would be this: *damage limitation*. It's about helping you keep the emotional rollercoaster on the tracks until you hit the flat bit, so you can both get off and back on your feet – instead of staying braced for the next nerve-shredding twist neither of you saw coming.

> **Instant expert**
>
> **Lucy Cavendish on keeping your relationship on the right track**
>
> *Lucy Cavendish is a relationships counsellor and author of* How to Have Extraordinary Relationships.[1] *She's worked with countless couples blindsided by menopause, helping them reconnect, communicate and come out stronger (www.lucycavendishlovecoach.com).*

Put yourself in her shoes

Society has long tied a woman's value to her fertility and desirability. Historically, post-menopausal women were sidelined or even cast out as withered old 'hags' or 'crones'. Today, those labels may not exist in the same way, but the underlying societal attitudes still linger. Even if she isn't consciously thinking like that, the shift away from fertility can impact her identity. She may be grappling with feelings of invisibility, grief and uncertainty about her future role. For some, menopause comes with a sense of relief. For others, there's a deep sense of loss.

Menopause is an opportunity, not a threat

A lot of men tell me that they used to have a good marriage but don't know what they did wrong – or what they can do about it. They think their marriage is over. But it's often not about them – it's about the menopause. They need to understand that their partners aren't the same people anymore. But neither of them is the same person their partner fell in love with. People change – physically, emotionally and psychologically – over time. Instead of lamenting these changes, get curious about who your partner now is. Ultimately, what gets couples through menopause isn't just information – it's empathy, patience, and the willingness to rediscover each other and evolve together.

Accept that this is really freaking hard

Going through 'the change' is still used to describe typical perimenopause symptoms, but it's important to remember it's not a quick or temporary shift; it's a fundamental biological and emotional transformation. On top of all this, hormonal changes often coincide with other major life transitions: children leaving home, ageing parents, possible career changes, and maybe even other personal health issues. It's a perfect storm of emotional and physical upheaval. The fear that things will never improve is overwhelming, but the reality is that, while menopause is a very challenging transition, it's not a new state of permanent misery.

Men need support, too

Davina McCall, Dr Louise Newson and others are doing incredible work in raising menopause awareness, but they primarily engage female audiences. This is one of the biggest unspoken challenges. Men often feel excluded from the dialogue and lack spaces to express their feelings. They think they're not allowed to say things like they don't recognize their partner anymore, or can't admit they don't know how to handle things – because if they speak up they fear being chastised and told, 'It's alright for you – you're not the one going through it.'

But men do need support. You need to be able to ask questions, share experiences, and navigate your feelings without judgement. You need to know you're not alone, either, and that there are ways to support your partner while also taking care of yourself.

Dangerous liaisons: Keeping cool when she can't

Just because you can now put yourself in her shoes doesn't mean she'll want – or be able – to step into yours. Not while she's drowning in hormonal chaos and still doesn't know which way's up.

There's a good chance you'll face some seriously testing moments: a sarcastic dig here, a cutthroat complaint there, and more than a few acidic accusations that put your love, loyalty … and manhood under serious scrutiny.

When that happens – and it will – don't explain, justify or caveat. You already know that's the shortcut to a full-blown row.

So what should you do? Tell her you understand and ask how you can help? Nope. Still wrong – at this stage, anyway. We'll get to that in the next chapter.

For now, there's only one goal: let her vent. Why? Because that's the fastest way to help her calm down.

'Sometimes, women don't want an answer. They don't want a solution. They just want their partner to sit with them in the feeling,' says sex and relationship expert Sarah Louise Ryan. We'll hear more from Sarah in Chapter 12, when we crack the code on reigniting passion, intimacy and sex (told you we'd cover all the bases).

Real talk

'I thought my wife was going mad – I had no idea what to do'

I'm Kevin. I'm 65 and a retired bank manager living in Edinburgh.

> If I'm honest, I knew nothing about any of this before it happened to Jane. I assumed that after her periods stopped there'd be a short amount of time when things were up in the air, then it would be over. A few months. A year at most. I couldn't believe it when it actually started and what was happening. When she said perimenopause could last for years, my heart sank. I didn't know how I'd get through it.
>
> We never really argued as such, but problems came out of nowhere, fast. One time I was painting the front room. She loved the colour and was really happy. But then she just snapped, making a massive deal out of a few flecks of stray paint. It was these instant changes in her character that completely threw me. One day she might tell me not to go near her; the next she'd be complaining I never gave her any attention. It's enough to make your head spin.

Stay strong – don't take the bait

So, this isn't about fixing – it's about feeling. When things get spiky, don't take it personally. It's stress, fear and frustration grabbing the wheel – not her deepest truth. She's not angling for a row. She just wants to be heard and noticed.

This section isn't about absorbing everything she says, decoding what's really behind it, or being a complete pushover. It's about not making things worse. Damage limitation, remember?

Here are five of the classic midlife flashpoints: what she might suddenly say, what's really going on underneath – and how not to respond if you want to avoid turning a spark into a full-blown inferno.

'I'm doing this all myself'

You might also hear: *You don't care about me, I do everything for everyone, No one ever helps me out.*

What's really up? She probably feels exhausted, isolated and invisible.

Don't ... tell her she should have just asked for help – she already has, in a hundred different ways.

What can you do? Right now? Suck it up. Then, as soon as the storm passes, start doing more – without waiting to be asked.

'You never listen to me'

You might also hear: *You're not here for me, You just don't get it, You're not even paying attention.*

What's really up? She's feeling emotionally dismissed and disconnected – and desperate to be heard.

Don't ... pretend you've no idea what she's on about, or reel off a few half-baked examples of why she's wrong.

What can you do? Stop. Listen. Maintain eye contact. Let her speak without interrupting – she won't stay mad for ever (just nod occasionally so your silence doesn't accidentally prove her point).

'All you care about is yourself'

You might also hear: *You just coast through life, You have no idea what it's like, You wouldn't last a day in my shoes.*

What's really up? She's overwhelmed, unsupported, and resenting how detached you seem from her day-to-day struggles.

Don't ... say you do understand, or start comparing stress levels – unless you want to turn a crack into a chasm.

What can you do? Tell her she's right – that you've not been pulling your weight (even if you think you have). Then let her know things are going to change from now on.

'I feel so ugly'

You might also hear: *I hate my body, You don't fancy me anymore, I want the old me back.*

What's really up? Her self-esteem has hit rock bottom – physically, emotionally, sexually – and she sees no way to bounce back.

Don't ... tell her she's being ridiculous or brush it off with, 'What are you talking about? You look fine.'

What can you do? Tell her something you genuinely find beautiful about her – and really mean it.

'I can't do this anymore'

You might also hear: *We're broken and I think I'm done, Too much has changed, I don't even recognize us anymore.*

What's really up? She's confused, scared, and grieving the loss of who she was – and what you had together.

Don't ... panic, argue or try to talk her out of it. This isn't a debate – it's a last-gasp cry for help.

What can you do? Be vulnerable. Tell her you're struggling with everything, too – and the one thing you want is to find a way through this together.

Anger management 101

How to defuse before you detonate

You're not a monster. You're not broken. You're just wired like every other human running the standard-issue stress response – the same one that kept our ancestors alive when they still ran up trees to escape predators.

Here's the deal: anger isn't just an emotion – it's a full-body chain reaction. It's part of your biological stress system, usually a manifestation of the fight in the fight–flight–freeze response – your body's primal alarm that gears you up to confront, escape or shut down when threatened.[2]

When your amygdala – the brain's threat detector – picks up something it doesn't like (probably not an apex carnivore, but a barbed comment, a slammed door, or a sudden shift in tone), it sets off the alarm. First comes adrenaline (aka epinephrine), which spikes your heart rate, blood pressure and breathing. Blood is directed away from low-priority jobs like digestion and straight to your muscles, prepping you for action. Then comes cortisol, the heavyweight stress hormone, which puts your brain on high alert (see Chapter 9).[3]

If you don't intervene, the surge peaks and hijacks your behaviour. Your prefrontal cortex, the rational, self-regulating part of your brain, goes offline.[4] And that's when you say or do something you later regret.

Getting ahead of anger

Here's the good news: this surge builds in stages – and, at each stage, you've got a small window to step in.[5] Spot the signs early (shallow breathing, clenched jaw, rising heat) and you can use calming strategies to short-circuit the cycle. These help trigger your parasympathetic nervous system – shifting you from high-alert fight–flight–freeze to the opposite state: calm, composed rest-and-digest.[6]

> The problem? In midlife, your system's already running hot. Stress, poor sleep, hormones and mental load crank up your baseline tension.[7] Add a shorter fuse and lower emotional bandwidth,[8] and you're far more likely to misread neutral cues – an innocent question, a raised eyebrow, an unexpected request – as a personal attack on your competence or character.
>
> The result? More frequent flare-ups and more explosive ones.
>
> But here's the truth: you're not trying to eliminate anger – that's impossible. It's about remembering that you can intervene. You do have influence. And in the heat of the moment, as soon as you clock what's happening, you're already back in control.

The deactivation dozen: How to buy time before you blow your top

Even with the best will in the world, there'll be something that's said or done that sets you off.

Suddenly you're seconds from exploding. Your jaw's tight, your fists are clenched, and you're breathing like you've just smashed a 5K PB. But blowing up never helps, and it makes everything worse for the next few hours, days or longer.

Next time, try these 12 science-backed strategies to give yourself a moment to let the red mist lift. No chakra chanting. No power poses. No airy-fairy philosophy – just fast, functional hacks to get your head straight before you say something you'll regret.

1 The sigh reset

Take two short inhales through your nose, then one long, slow exhale through your mouth.

Why? Known as the 'physiological sigh', it rapidly lowers your heart rate and tells your nervous system to stand down.[9]

2 Box breathing

Inhale for four seconds, hold for four, exhale for four, hold again for four – then repeat.

Why? Breathwork slows your heart and breathing rate, calms your nervous system, and gives your brain time to respond rather than react[10] (see Chapter 9).

3 Counting to 10

Silently count from 1 to 10 at a steady pace.

Why? It's old-school, but it works – it delays knee-jerk reactions by giving your brain a vital pause.[11]

4 Label the feeling

In your mind give a name to what you're feeling, like 'This is anger' or 'This is pain'.

Why? Naming emotions takes out the sting: it separates your reaction from their action to put you in control of the feeling, so it stops controlling you.[12]

5 Change the channel

Mentally name all the countries you've visited, list your top five TV shows, or recite the lyrics of your favourite song.

Why? Distraction works like a circuit breaker – it forces your brain to switch tracks and stops you spiralling.[13]

6 Pick a positive phrase

Repeat a meaningful mantra like 'Let it go' or 'I've got this'.

Why? Positive words drown out the mental noise and refocus your mindset.[14]

7 Clench and release your fists

Squeeze your fists tightly for five seconds, then slowly release. (Best done in your pockets.)

Why? It resets your grip on the moment – literally – so you don't lose your grip emotionally.[15]

8 Change your posture

Drop your shoulders, release your jaw, and loosen your hands.

Why? Relaxed body language sends calming signals to your brain and shows others you're not on the attack.[16]

9 Move your muscles

Any kind of movement works: stand, stretch, pace or shake everything out.

Why? Movement burns off pent-up stress-fuel and tells your brain the danger's over.[17]

10 Splash cold water

Splash your face or run ice-cold water over your hands and wrists.

Why? It activates the dive reflex – a calming response that slows your heart and pulls you out of fight-or-flight mode.[18]

11 Call a time-out

Step away and take a few minutes to breathe.

Why? Super simple: a short break stops the spiral and gives both of you space to cool off.[19]

12 Ground your senses

Name five things you see, four you feel, three you hear, two you smell and one you taste.

Why? This 5-4-3-2-1 method brings you out of your head and back into the moment ... fast.[20]

It's time to talk and turn things around

You've learned how to stay calm in the chaos. Now it's time to take the next step and actually talk about what's going on.

Because, however bad things might feel right now, they don't have to stay that way. It's rarely a lack of love that drives couples apart at this stage of life – it's a lack of understanding of what the other person is really going through, and a lack of practical know-how on how to help.

This is the turning point. You've seen the problem from all sides – so now we move towards the solutions. You know what's going on – with you, with her, with your relationship – and it's time to do something with that knowledge. That means talking. In the next chapter, we'll show you how – including what to say, what not to say, and how to have the conversations that can change everything.

Some of these talks might be the hardest of your life. But that's OK. The hardest conversations are usually the ones you've been avoiding. Once they start, everything else can start to fall into place.

6

Breaking the ice
How to talk without making things worse

You're through the emotional storm, the red mist has lifted, and you kept your head – even if no one else did. Now it's time to talk. The trouble? Words don't always come easy – not when the air is thick with the unspoken reality of what no one has managed to say out loud. Yet.

Soon you'll have the tools and tactics to start the conversations that matter. You'll learn how to listen better, side-step conversational quicksand, and really get through to one another. Not with a perfect script but with enough awareness to turn emotional chaos into mutual understanding.

In this chapter you'll discover:

- The golden rules that stop important conversations from going south
- How to pick the right time and place for tough talks
- Why silence is your secret superpower and how to use it right
- The exact words and phrases that shut her down and what to say instead
- How to ask questions that make her open up, not feel interrogated
- What your body language is really saying and how to change the message
- Smart ways to defuse arguments, repair connection and bounce back stronger
- The fun game to decode each other's emotional turn-ons and turn-offs.

By now, you've started to make sense of what's been happening. To her. To you. Maybe it felt like trying to crack two separate codes, only to realize they're part of the same puzzle.

What happens next? That depends on you. Because insight is just the beginning. Real change only happens when you start talking about the stuff that matters. That's not easy – especially when it's tangled up with guilt, shame, confusion, embarrassment, and all the feelings you've both been keeping under wraps for weeks or months.

The trouble is dodging hard conversations doesn't protect your relationship – it risks tearing it apart. But once you know how to talk? Everything shifts. Not overnight. But when the stakes feel this high, every small win is a big step forward.

The 10 golden rules of better conversations

Before we reveal how to level up your communication skills, we need to cover the conversational booby traps – the reasons so many chats go tits up before they've really started.

These are the unspoken ground rules that make or break your relationship. Get them right and you're halfway there. Get them wrong? You're back to square one: silence, sulking and sleeping on the sofa.

1 **Most fights don't come out of nowhere.** They build over time – through background tension, passive-aggressive comments or weeks of simmering frustration. What feels like a sudden explosion is usually the end of a long, flickering fuse.
2 **The hardest thing to say is what's going on.** It's really hard to admit you're not coping, especially when you don't know why. It's much easier to go quiet or lash out than admit how you feel. Most arguments between couples aren't about what was just said or done – they're about what wasn't.
3 **The hardest thing to hear? The truth.** The truth hurts: especially if she's been denying it – to you, herself or everyone else. That's why blunt accusations backfire. But patience, empathy and open-ended questions give her the space to say what she's struggling to admit.
4 **Most people take things at face value.** If she says, 'I'm fine', it's easy to assume she is. But 'fine' can mean sad. Or furious. Or simply too tired to say anything more. Learning to read between the lines – and spotting body language signs – is invaluable.

5. **Her body will tell you more than her words.** Raised shoulders. Clenched fists. Arms crossed. If something about her body language feels stiff, tense or stressed, then so is she – no matter what she says.
6. **When and where you talk makes a big difference.** Face-to-face conversations can feel like confrontations and shut things down fast. Side-by-side chats are the way to go. And don't dive into anything deep and meaningful when you're both tired and distracted (see below).
7. **Trying to 'win' the conversation? You've already lost.** When you're angry, frustrated or desperate, you want to defend yourself, get a confession or prove a point. But this isn't a debate – it's a dialogue. It's not about winning, it's about understanding. If your ego's driving, you're headed for a crash.
8. **One good talk won't fix everything.** This isn't Hollywood. You're not going to have 'the chat', cry it out, rip each other's clothes off, then skip off into the sunset. Real change takes consistency. And that requires empathy, patience and – crucially – time.
9. **The calmest voice sets the tone.** In every exchange, someone determines the tempo. If you stay steady, grounded and kind, you give her the option to follow suit. That's not your weakness. That's how you both win.
10. **You will get it wrong – so own it.** You'll say the wrong thing, pick the wrong time, or lose your temper. That's human. What matters is what happens next. A simple 'I got that wrong – can we try again?' can reset the whole mood. It shows you're listening, learning and really care about what's going on.

> **Forget trying to fix it!**
>
> This is your new mantra. When she opens up, don't jump in with a fix. Even if it sounds like the perfect solution, that's not what she needs. Your job is to keep the space open so she can talk for as long as she needs.

The right time and place to talk

When and where you talk can be as important as what you say, yet hardly anyone gives it a second thought. And that's often the first – and biggest – mistake. Here's how to get it right.

The right moment

Pick the wrong moment – when one of you is exhausted, distracted, stressed or already upset – and even the best intentions can backfire fast. Avoid early mornings (when you're still coming round), late nights (when you're trying to wind down), or five minutes before someone needs to be somewhere. A ticking clock adds pressure you don't need. If it feels rushed or emotionally charged, it's not the right time. Not sure when to talk? First choose the right setting.

The right location

Never sit face to face – this isn't a job interview. That kind of formal setup adds intensity, pressure and judgement. Go shoulder to shoulder instead. A walk, a long drive, peeling potatoes at the sink – something that gets you physically aligned. When your body language says, 'We're in this together' and not 'We're squaring off', there's less confrontation and more honesty, and the words come more easily.

The right routine

The best way to get timing and location right? Make it a habit. Find regular moments in your week where conversation comes naturally – a morning walk, a coffee break, or lunch out with no phones in sight. Regular chats release steam little and often, so pressure doesn't build until someone blows up. When talking becomes routine, even the hardest conversations stop feeling like a ticking time bomb.

> **Instant expert**
>
> **Nigel Taberner on turning conflict into compassion**
>
> *Nigel Taberner is a former hostage negotiator who spent decades resolving stand-offs, de-escalating danger and talking people back*

from the brink. He believes his approach to calm, respectful communication isn't just for crisis situations: it's exactly what men need to build trust, manage emotions and make life easier – even during the most challenging times (nigeltaberner.com).

Silence is your secret weapon

When men feel uncomfortable, they talk. We try to explain, justify or fix things before we've even understood the problem. But over-talking shuts the other person down and ramps up tension. In a standoff, one wrong word can escalate everything. I learned fast that silence isn't a gap to be filled – it's an invaluable tool. Let her speak without interruption. Resist the urge to jump in. Stay quiet and present. It shows her you're not trying to control the conversation – just understand her.

Questions are never the answer

In tense moments, most men become interrogators: 'What's wrong?' 'What did I do?' 'What do you need?' But questions can feel like pressure, especially if your tone or timing is off. Early in my career, I learned to reflect instead of probe. If she says, 'I've had a nightmare day', don't quiz her: reflect it, 'You've had a nightmare day?' It shows you're listening and invites her to keep going – in her own time. If that feels odd, try open-ended phrases like 'Tell me more about it'.

Stop saying you understand – you don't

One of the biggest mistakes men make is rushing to relate. Saying 'I understand' might feel supportive, but it rarely lands well – especially when the other person is overwhelmed, angry or confused. That one phrase shuts people down faster than anything else. It makes them feel unheard or brushed aside. A better approach is to admit it: 'I can't imagine what that's like – but I want to understand.' That creates safety. You're not downplaying her experience – you're making space for it.

Keep your head to keep control

In every high-pressure situation I've faced, one truth always holds: the person who stays composed holds the advantage. That doesn't mean staying flat or robotic. When someone's emotion spikes, you don't mirror their anger, but you do need to meet their intensity in a way that shows you understand this matters to them. If you stay completely calm while they escalate, the disconnect can actually make things worse. Matching energy – without matching emotion – helps maintain connection and de-escalate tension. It's not easy, but it's essential.

Always give her a way out

When tension builds, don't push harder or raise your voice. If someone feels cornered, they'll fight. One of the most effective strategies in a crisis is offering someone a dignified way out. At home, that might sound like: 'Maybe now's not the best time – but I'm here when you're ready.' The best conversations happen only when both people feel calm and in control – not cornered.

What to say – and what not to

Getting someone who doesn't want to talk to open up can feel like trying to crack a safe with a stick of celery. A concerned 'Are you OK?' gets a clipped 'I'm fine'. You ask again and get your head bitten off. So you back away – only later to be accused of not giving a damn.

It's a simplification, sure, but the vibe might resonate. So what the hell should you do?

Ask better questions. What you ask, how you phrase it, and the tone you use can either build a bridge or burn it down. Here's how to avoid conversational quicksand, sidestep landmine language, and start talking more honestly – and more often.

How to ask the right questions

The questions we ask often reveal more about us than the other person. When you say, 'Are you OK?', it's usually code for 'Please tell me everything's fine so I can go and play golf'. And that's exactly what she hears.

The real trick to kick off a positive conversation is to lower the pressure – not raise it. That means ditching interrogation-style or dead-end yes-or-no questions for ones that give her the space to have a proper swing, like:

'You don't seem quite yourself – want to talk?'
'Can you describe how you're feeling? I really want to understand.'
'I get the sense I've said something that landed badly?'

'I'm sensing I've missed something, haven't I?'
'It seems like something's bothering you – is that fair?'

Reflect, don't redirect

Non-judgemental phrases like these are conversation starters, not stoppers. But what if she says something vague or confusing like 'I just feel really off'?

Try reflecting it back: 'You feel off?' Bouncing it back encourages her to keep talking without making her feel interrogated. There's no pressure – you're proving you're present.

Remember, your job isn't to solve, it's to understand. And even if you think you do, don't say it out loud. Why?

One, you almost certainly don't understand. You may feel tired, stressed or anxious, too, but chances are you know what's causing it. She probably doesn't. That's the difference.

Two, don't relate it back to you. Saying something like 'I know exactly what it's like – my mum went through menopause' may feel helpful and supportive, but it's not. It hijacks the moment, steals her spotlight, and undermines her unique experience. Instead, try something like:

'I can't pretend to understand what this feels like, but tell me.'
'It sounds like you're carrying a lot right now.'
'I get the impression you've been feeling like this for a while.'

The aim is simple: your turn in the conversation has one job – to make it her turn again.

Active listening 101

How to really hear what she's saying

Most people think they're great listeners.[1] Most of the time they're just waiting for the chance to start talking. Active listening is different. It's not about jumping in with solutions or dropping a perfectly timed hot take. It's about making the other person feel seen, heard and safe so they keep talking. Here's how to do it.

1. **Listen to understand, not to respond.** The best listeners are detectives, not debaters. Don't drift off to rehearse your perfect comment or comeback. Stay curious. Listen closely. Follow her lead.
2. **Take your time to reply.** Silence can feel awkward, but pausing before you speak shows you were really listening and gives her the chance to keep going.
3. **Use your eyes, not just your ears.** Look for hunched shoulders, clenched jaw, crossed arms, restless movements or sudden silence. Because what she's feeling might not come out in words, but it's written all over her body.
4. **Recap in her words.** Once she's got it off her chest, play it back using her own words to check you've understood. Either you have – great! – or she'll go deeper.
5. **Match her energy, not her emotion.** If she's fired up, don't go cold. If she's quiet, don't come in loud. Tune into her intensity, not her mood – it shows you're present and encourages her to keep going.
6. **Say 'Thanks for telling me'.** End with appreciation, not advice. Even if the conversation was heavy or messy, those four words validate the risk she took in sharing and make it more likely she'll open up again.
7. **Lose the pressure to be perfect.** Follow the rest of this list and you don't need to be perfect. If you stay present and really listen, you've given her what she needed most.

Keep her talking

Once she starts to open up, the last thing you want to do is shut her down, but even kind, well-meaning words can do it. Take this example:

> HER: 'I'm just tired of doing it all.'
> YOU: 'You are? I'm sorry.'

It sounds supportive, but you've stalled the conversation instead of shifting it up a gear. Instead try:

> 'You're dealing with too much right now.'
> 'I'm not here to fix it – I'm here to hear it. Talk to me.'
> 'If I'm quiet, it's because I'm listening – not because I don't care.'

It's a subtle difference, but it keeps the focus on her and demonstrates she's being heard. That can be enough to make her keep going.

Will you get it wrong? Absolutely. Probably many times. But that's fine. Say, 'I'm not sure I've handled this well – can we start over?' That shows you care. Mistakes might even help. If you say, 'You sound angry,' and she replies, 'No, I'm just exhausted,' you're learning something. Now you can get back on track – 'It seems like you're spread far too thin right now' – to coax her to say more.

Real talk

'Learning to listen might save your marriage'

I'm Jaz. I'm 54 and I live in Milton Keynes. I'm a resilience expert, multiple award-winning international speaker and author of Because of You, This is Me: The Stories We Tell, The Stories We Change and the Power of Everyday Heroes.[2] *I've trained teachers, starred in TV shows, and built my whole identity around being the strong one who always knows what to say. But when I couldn't find the words to tell my husband what I needed, we came up with a simple shorthand – and it changed everything (jazampawfarr.com).*

'Communication has been the one thing that's made the biggest difference in my marriage to Ed. In the early days, when it felt like there was no way through, it was because of a lack of it. If we've celebrated, it's been because of clear communication. It's made us – and saved us – more than once.

Everyone has different natural modes of communication, and figuring those out can make all the difference. For me, my default is celebration. Sometimes I want care. Less often, I want critique. What I need changes – it depends on what kind of day I'm having.

So Ed will say, 'Do you want celebration, care, or critique right now?' It sounds simple, but that one question has changed everything. I don't feel like he's trying to fix me or shut me down. He's letting me lead – and then giving me what I need.

Listening is a big one, too, and I don't always want a conversation. Some mornings, I wake up with 6,000 ideas and I'll say, 'Can you come and talk to me while I'm in the shower?' I don't actually need him to say a word. I just need him to be there, listening. He'll raise his

> eyebrows, nod or say 'Mmm' at the right time. I know he's listening and holding back answering my hypothetical questions!
>
> All he's doing is being there, being with me, and it makes me feel so loved. That kind of presence – not fixing, not freaking out, just standing beside me – has pulled us back from the edge more than once. I genuinely think that's why we're still married – because of his commitment to 'withness'.

The power of language and tone

So yes, what you say really matters, but words are only a small part of communication.[3]

Humans are hardwired to detect threat.[4] That includes changes in tone, pitch, posture and energy. You can pick the right words, but if the delivery is defensive, dismissive or disinterested, she'll know it and shut down before you've finished your sentence. So what does calm and safe delivery actually mean?

Lower your voice slightly. Don't mumble but bring the volume down a notch. You're not broadcasting. You're inviting.

Speak slowly. Not robotic. Just enough to show you're in control of your emotions. Rushed speech = rattled mind.

Soften your stance. Arms uncrossed. Jaw unclenched. Body angled slightly towards her. These cues show you're calm – so she won't feel cornered.

Use your hands. Keep them relaxed and open. Avoid pointing or fist clenching. A palms-up gesture shows openness and trust.

Really mean it. If your words say, 'I'm listening', but your face says, 'If we stop now I can catch the second half', it will land like a slap in the face. Authenticity matters most.

Conversation killers 101

The danger lines that kill your connection

Some words seem harmless. Others sound supportive. But even when they're well-meaning, certain phrases can kill connection stone dead. Here are the worst offenders:

'Calm down.' Nothing triggers defensiveness faster and no one has ever calmed down because they were told to. But you knew this already, right?

'You're overreacting.' The fastest way to make someone feel small – and shut them down for the foreseeable.

'You always ...' or 'You never ...' These two turn a specific issue into a full-blown character assassination. Now you're not talking about what's just happened – you're fighting about everything, ever.

'You just need to ...' Sounds helpful. Feels dismissive, patronizing and arrogant all at once. She doesn't need a fix – she wants to be heard. Focus on empathy, not action points.

'But I've had a tough day, too.' Now it's a competition. You've yanked the spotlight back to you and turned her vulnerability into a point-scoring game where even if you win, you lose.

'You've been like this for weeks.' It might be true, but it's loaded with blame. And it doesn't matter – what does is that you're finally talking.

'I didn't mean it like that.' Now you're arguing about your intention instead of owning the impact. You don't get to decide how your words land – she does.

'I'm just being honest.' Always code for, 'I'm about to say something blunt and don't want to be held responsible'. Honesty without empathy isn't brave – it's cruel.

'That's not how I see it.' It might be your truth, but that's not the point. The goal isn't to be right – it's to understand what she's feeling and why.

When it all starts going south

You've now got a grip on what to say and how to say it. But some days it might feel like you're stuck in *Squid Game* – one wrong move and it's game over.

Tough chats can spiral fast when emotions have been simmering for a while, tempers are frayed, and fear or frustration have been bubbling just beneath the surface for longer than either of you realized.

The good news? A few smart tactics can keep you in the game.

Go in with a game plan

Every conversation is better when you don't wing it. You don't need to script every word, but spending a couple of minutes to clarify what you want to achieve, and what might get in the way, can make all the difference. Here's how:

- **Know your aim.** Are you hoping to understand how she's really doing or to open up about what's going on with you? Either way, your goal is the same: create enough space, time and safety for real feelings to surface.
- **Think small.** Whether you're dreaming of recapturing your honeymoon phase or simply stop snapping at each other, you won't solve it in one go. Sometimes the most productive chat is the one that gets things moving – not the one that wraps everything up.
- **Anticipate the roadblocks.** What's likely to come up? What's derailed conversations before? What's she likely to say that will trigger you, and how can you keep your cool in that moment?
- **Stay grounded.** Emotions start in the body, not the brain. The calmer you are going in, the better you'll handle what happens next. Drop your shoulders. Loosen your jaw. Breathe slower. You could even try a quick calming breath exercise (see Chapter 9).

Instant expert

Jessica Barac on the communication shortcuts that save the day

Jessica Barac is a registered nutritionist, personal trainer and founder of What The Menopause, a global women's health platform. After struggling to get answers during her own perimenopause, she made it her mission to crack the menopause code and help other women feel strong, stable and sexy (whatthemenopause.com).

Forget mind-reading – try code words

There are days when explaining how we feel is impossible. A shared shorthand really helps with damage control. Start with simple concepts. Using colours – for example 'I'm on red today' for rage, or blue for sadness – works brilliantly. Or try battery levels: 'I'm running at 20 percent.' It lets her flag high-emotion or low-capacity days without a full backstory, and gets you on the same team instantly.

Ask the question that matters

You want to help, but most of the time you guess. And it's easy to guess wrong. Instead try, 'Do you want to be hugged, helped or heard?' It may sound silly, but it cuts straight through. Some days we want advice. Some days a cuddle. Some days we just want to be seen. Asking instead of assuming means we both win.

Silence doesn't mean we're fine

At my lowest, I didn't talk. I didn't have the words. So if she's gone quiet, don't probe, but don't vanish either. Say, 'I'm here when you're ready.' Then back it up. Stay close. Be visible. We need to know we're not alone.

Don't take the bite at face value

Yes, we'll snap. We'll cry. We'll rage. And yes, we'll take it out on you. But nine times out of ten, it's not about what we're shouting about – it's about everything we're holding in. Stay calm and say, 'This isn't like you – what's really going on?' You'll defuse the moment and help her open up.

One chat won't fix it, but showing up will

There were times I couldn't even ask for help. I just wanted someone to say, 'I see you. I hear you. You're not going mad.' I didn't get that. But it taught me this: you don't need to be perfect. Just show up. Be there. That's what builds trust. Not one big conversation – but being present again and again, even in the chaos.

When the shit hits the fan

Sometimes, as we touched on in Chapter 5, even when you've followed the plan to perfection, she might blow up out of nowhere. There's nothing you could've done differently, and she might not even know why she's swinging between red-hot fury and sudden tears. It could be months of anger finally boiling over or the sheer overwhelm of finally talking about what's going on.

But you don't need to know why. You need to ride out the storm.

Former police negotiator Nigel Taberner – who we met earlier in this chapter – says the golden rule in any high-stakes situation is simple: buy yourself time. Why? Because no one can stay angry for ever. Extreme emotion is exhausting – physically and mentally – and it can't be sustained. Especially if she feels like she's being heard. Here's what to do:

- **Let her vent.** Interrupting mid-flow only shortens the fuse.
- **Use silence.** A short pause after she's finished gives her space to breathe and you time to respond.
- **Reflect, don't react.** Bounce it back to show you're listening. 'I've clearly misunderstood something here – can you help me get it right?'

You don't need to agree. But you must listen. That's enough to dial down the temperature so you both can regroup.

If all else fails, give her a way out

In the heat of the moment, people say things they don't mean. If you call it out, she might double down – it's hard to admit you were out of line, especially when you want to 'win' the conversation.

The smarter move? Give her a lifeline, not a lecture. It's another strategy from hostage negotiation – giving someone the chance to back down with their head held high.

So reframe the comment with warmth or humour, not blame or sarcasm. It's not about ignoring what was said. It's about pressing pause, letting things cool down, and resuming the conversation without anyone feeling cornered or ashamed.

Try sentences like:

'Let's not make this about that one comment – what's really going on here?'

'It sounds like there's more underneath this. I'd rather get to that than get into a row.'

'We've both said things under pressure before. I'd rather understand than score points.'

'This doesn't feel like the real issue – can we hit pause and figure it out together?'

'Let's take five and get some air – I could do with a change of scenery.'

'Should we take a timeout and have a coffee? Might help us both clear our heads.'

Responses like this show you're not here to win, punish or prove a point – you're here to protect the space between you. Because that's how trust is built – not in the calm or carefree moments, but in how you handle the hard ones.

The traffic light list of dos and don'ts

Every couple has their little flashpoints: tiny things that seem completely innocuous to you yet have an uncanny ability to make her giddy with love … or incandescent with rage. And it works both ways. You might have no idea that leaving your socks on the floor makes her blood boil. She might not realize that repeatedly asking what's happening in a movie you're watching for the first time together drives you insane. Yet some couples never discover the easy wins to their partner's heart – or the petty patterns that quietly build resentment.

Lights, clarity, action

The traffic light list is a quick and fun way to figure out what makes each other tick, so you can do more of the things that make her feel loved – and less of what makes her wish she had a voodoo doll of you in her knicker drawer.

Don't overthink it. Don't justify. Don't caveat. Just write it down then swap notes. Start with green, then amber, then red. And remember, this isn't about blame. It's about giving each other a cheat sheet for more joy, less stress and the occasional chest-puffing 'I nailed that' moment.

And yes, you can even do a bedroom version of your green list as a shortcut to rekindling romance. Here's how it works:

Green = I love it when you …

These are the small, meaningful gestures that fill the tank. Maybe it's bringing her a coffee in the morning, a WhatsApp check-in when she's up against it, or booking a surprise dinner at her favourite restaurant. These are your easy wins – do them often.

Amber = It's jarring when you …

These are the grey areas. Checking your phone during dinner. Not asking if she needs anything before you go shopping. Never replacing the loo roll. They're not deal-breakers, but catch her at the wrong moment, or do it too often, and it is a big deal.

Red = For the love of God, don't ever …

These are the emotional landmines – the things that make her feel invisible, unheard or totally unimportant. Leaving the kitchen a mess after she's cleaned it. Hijacking her stories because you 'tell them better'. Forgetting to pick up the kid/cat/cousin from the school/vet/airport, even though she reminded you 20 times. These are the moments that make her start googling divorce lawyers.

Keep showing up

Now you know how to ask better questions, really listen to her answers, and stop conversations spiralling into sulks, standoffs and slammed doors.

You're not here to fix her. You're here to face it with her. And that shift in mindset – from pressure to partnership – changes everything.

It shows her she's not alone and proves that, even when the conversation turns cold, you're prepared to figure it out together.

That matters. Not just for her – for both of you.

Because as you'll discover in the next chapter, perimenopause isn't just a physical journey. It's an emotional rollercoaster, and there'll be many white-knuckle days ahead. But you've already done the hardest bit: you've started talking. Just keep doing it – everything gets easier if you do.

7

Dealing with the doctor
Making sure she's taken seriously

You've backed her from the sidelines. Now it's time to stand shoulder to shoulder and help her get the support she deserves. We'll give you the know-how to help her access the right care – whether that's through the NHS, a private clinic or an online provider. You'll learn when it's time to book the appointment, what to do before, during and after, and how to avoid getting the dreaded brush-off.

The healthcare system isn't always kind or consistent. It can be slow, frustrating, and full of dead ends. But with you by her side, she won't have to face it alone.

In this chapter you'll discover:
- The eight warning signs she needs medical support
- What to do before, during and after her appointment
- How to help her avoid being misdiagnosed or dismissed
- How to tell if a doctor is worth their salt – or wasting her time
- What to expect from public, private and online healthcare
- How to support her every step of the way.

Let's be honest: no one likes going to the doctor. It's never a fun way to spend a morning – unless you've got a thing for fluorescent lighting and five-year-old magazines. But if she's struggling with her symptoms, she may need to see a medical professional.

Yet here's the rub: getting the right help is rarely straightforward. In many countries, including the UK, basic menopause training isn't standard. In fact, 41 percent of UK medical schools don't include mandatory menopause education.[1] The outcome? Many women are often dismissed, misdiagnosed or sent packing with nothing but platitudes and paracetamol.

The US – where healthcare access depends on what you can afford – is no better: fewer than one in five obstetrician-gynaecologists (OB-GYNs) receive formal training in how to support women through menopause.[2] And around the world, outdated concerns about hormone replacement therapy (HRT – see Chapter 8) still prevent millions of women from getting the safe, effective and evidence-based treatment that could really help.[3]

Different systems, same outcome

Women in perimenopause and menopause are being let down. Not because they're not trying hard enough but because most healthcare systems aren't designed to support them.

And that's where you come in – with the curiosity to understand and the courage to care. Because getting the right support isn't just about seeing the right doctor – it's about having someone beside her who won't let her go through this alone.

8 signs she needs to see a doctor

If she's been struggling for a while, it's hard on her and on you – especially if you feel powerless to make a difference. And that's OK. You're not expected to have the answers – even if you are a doctor, you're not *her* doctor – but you are in a unique position to help.

Because no matter how many hugs, hot baths or herbal teas you offer, she may need medical support. Here are the signs it's time to see someone with their own stethoscope ... and handwriting that looks like the heat map of a drunk spider on roller skates.

1. **Her symptoms are derailing daily life.** If hot flushes, night sweats, anxiety, brain fog, low mood, exhaustion or any other symptoms are interfering with her work, relationships or basic quality of life, it's time to get help. Perimenopause shouldn't make life unmanageable.
2. **Her emotional resilience has collapsed.** If anger and sadness are her constant companions, and tiny problems provoke big reactions, something's up. Seek help. Don't wait.
3. **Her body's playing up for no reason.** Heart palpitations, joint pain, headaches, gut issues, hair loss, bladder problems, itchy skin – when seemingly random physical complaints pile up, she needs advice. And don't settle if conventional tests come back 'normal' – ask for a menopause specialist (see below).
4. **Her sleep's a total mess.** If she's waking drenched in sweat or wide awake for hours every night, act now. Poor sleep ruins lives. She needs to break the cycle before it breaks her – and you.
5. **Lifestyle fixes are not touching the sides.** Exercise, good food, more sleep and less stress can all help – and we'll show you how in Chapters 9, 10 and 11 – but if she's too tired or overwhelmed to even think about healthier habits, she might need help to kickstart her comeback.
6. **She's under 45 and showing symptoms.** If she's under 45 – and especially under 40 – and showing signs like irregular periods, low mood or brain fog, don't wait it out.[4] Early or premature menopause needs proper investigation, treatment and care to protect long-term health.
7. **Her periods are very heavy or highly irregular.** Very heavy, erratic or prolonged periods are a classic sign of perimenopause,[5] but they can also point to other issues like fibroids or polyps.[6] If her cycle's changed dramatically, it's better to be safe than sorry.
8. **She's struggling with sexual health issues.** Vaginal dryness, pain during sex, low libido or bladder problems can be tough to talk about – but they're very common and often easily treated (see Chapter 8).[7,8] She shouldn't suffer in silence.

> **UK vs US healthcare**
>
> Live in the UK or a country with public healthcare? Keep reading for how to get the most from your GP or local health service. In the US or where private healthcare is the norm? Skip this section to find advice tailored to your country's system.

Instant expert

Dr Louise Newson on what GPs keep getting wrong

Dr Louise Newson is a GP, menopause specialist and best-selling author[9] whose work is transforming how women are diagnosed, treated and supported through perimenopause and menopause (drlouisenewson.co.uk). She's leading the charge to put better education, faster access and individualized care at the heart of menopause medicine.

Most doctors don't understand menopause

Medical schools barely cover menopause, and even specialist training like gynaecology focuses more on surgery and fertility than on recognizing perimenopausal and menopausal symptoms or treating them properly. So most GPs, gynaecologists and even endocrinologists finish training with only limited tuition on perimenopause and menopause, or how to prescribe HRT safely. That's why so many women are dismissed, misdiagnosed or wrongly treated – not because doctors don't care, but because they've never been taught.

Doctors treat the symptoms, not the cause

When women come in troubled by anxiety, low mood, insomnia or heart palpitations – common symptoms of perimenopause – they're often told they're just depressed or stressed or offered antidepressants. When hormone change is the root problem, hormone therapy is the first-line treatment in NICE guidance. But when doctors aren't taught to connect those symptoms to hormones, they end up treating each one in isolation. That means women suffer – when the right treatment could really help.

You can't trust blood tests

Hormone levels during perimenopause fluctuate so wildly that a blood test might show up as 'normal' even when symptoms are anything but. Blood tests only give a snapshot in time, not the full picture. NICE advises skipping blood tests altogether in women over 45 and basing diagnosis on symptoms, age and cycle changes. Relying on blood tests alone can delay treatment and leave women without the help they need.

Every woman's menopause looks different

There's no single set of symptoms. Some women have hot flushes and night sweats. Others never do, but struggle with memory lapses, low libido or crashing fatigue. These problems don't always seem hormonal at first. That's what makes diagnosis so hard. But the real issue is that we don't talk enough about how varied and widespread the symptoms can be. It's no wonder women doubt themselves. Just because she's not sweating through the night doesn't mean it's not her hormones. Always trust the symptoms – not the stereotypes.

Women have to fight hardest when they feel their worst

One of the cruellest realities of perimenopause is that it can strip away the very energy, clarity and confidence women need to stand up for themselves. I know this first-hand. Even though I was a menopause specialist, I was so exhausted, foggy and flat that I didn't recognize what was happening. Imagine how hard it is for women without the knowledge or support. When she's at her lowest ebb, she can't fight for the care she needs. That's why having a supportive partner – someone who believes her, backs her and keeps her going – can make all the difference.

Call the doctor and get the right result first time

As a man, your experience of seeing the doctor is probably straightforward. Got a sore throat? Book an appointment, get the once-over, get drugs. Job done.

But for women dealing with perimenopause, it's rarely that simple.

One in ten women has to attend between six and ten GP appointments before their symptoms are diagnosed as perimenopause or menopause, according to a survey of 6,000 women by Newson Health.[10]

Another survey – of over 5,000 women by menopause symptom-tracking app Balance – found that one in 14 women (7 percent) had to attend more than ten GP appointments before receiving adequate help or advice. Of those who eventually got treatment, only 37 percent were offered HRT – while 23 percent were prescribed antidepressants.[11]

That's despite guidance from NICE that says HRT should be the first-line treatment for menopause-related symptoms and that antidepressants should not be used for menopause-related low mood in most cases.[12] Yet 44 percent of women who receive HRT had to wait more than a year – and one in eight had waited over five years.[13]

That offer of HRT at the first appointment? Don't hold your breath.

Real talk

'My GP said I was depressed, but it was perimenopause'

I'm Jane. I'm 63, I'm a retired secretary, and I live on the Isle of Wight.

My first symptoms? A lack of sleep, brain fog and memory loss – I'd just forget things. It completely crushed my confidence. I'd have to write everything down. In my day-to-day life, working in a school, I had to get very good at putting strategies into place to cope. I had to adopt them at home, too – I was always making lists, then checking them twice. It was exhausting. And the hot flushes! The term doesn't do them justice! It's like I'm boiling from the inside. A surge of heat starts in my feet then flows up through my body. And it's rarely quick – some last for ages. At home I'll sit in my bra fanning myself with my top.

When I finally went to the GP he said it was depression, and gave me antidepressants. That took the edge off, but didn't really help me feel like myself again. He'd missed the clues about what was really going on – my brain fog, anxiety and depression were perimenopause playing out and it really affected my life.

After doing a lot of research myself, I saw another doctor and was prescribed HRT. Unfortunately, it was the wrong kind – I was given HRT for women still having periods, but mine had already completely stopped. So I saw another doctor and, after a lot of trial and error, was finally given the right treatment.

Gaslit by the GP: No tests, no treatment, no trust

When you don't know what's going on, there's little worse than finding the courage to seek help, only to be told you're making a mountain out of a molehill.

Medical gaslighting happens when a patient's symptoms are downplayed, dismissed or blamed on something else entirely – often stress, anxiety or 'just getting older'. It's especially common during perimenopause, when vague or variable symptoms are easily brushed aside.[14]

It's not just upsetting – it's dangerous. Being repeatedly told 'It's nothing' or 'Come back if it gets worse' delays diagnosis, treatment and relief. It undermines confidence and trust – not just in medical professionals but in herself.[15]

If she leaves an appointment feeling unheard, doubted or ashamed for raising the issue, that's not her fault. It's the system failing to meet her needs – and means it's time to start exploring other routes.

From roadblocks to results

Weeks, months, even years of uncertainty can cause untold stress and anxiety. She may feel overwhelmed, confused or fearful about what's happening – when safe and effective solutions are available.

The system doesn't make it easy: that's why it's crucial to have a plan to get the right result, ideally from her first GP appointment. Here's the four-step plan to ensure she gets the support she needs.

Step 1: When to book the appointment

Her symptoms are unrelenting

If her symptoms are affecting her daily life – constant anxiety, brain fog, exhaustion, insomnia, hot flushes or mood swings – don't wait for it to get any worse. The longer she struggles without medical support, the more overwhelmed and isolated she'll become. Insisting she's fine despite overwhelming evidence to the contrary? Going through the 'Eight signs she needs to see a doctor' list (see above) together may help her see the wood for the trees.

Healthier habits aren't cutting it

Lifestyle changes can make a big difference, and we'll show you how in Chapters 9, 10 and 11.

But sometimes willpower alone isn't enough. And she might not have the energy, clarity or confidence to even think about her habits right now, let alone change them. That's not a moral failure. It means she needs medical support to feel like herself again.

Ask for the right doctor

Once she's made the decision to go to the GP, ask if she can see someone who has experience in women's health or the menopause. Not all GPs have the same knowledge, training or – unfortunately – empathy. If not, a good GP will still listen, ask the right questions and suggest support options. What if they don't? Don't worry – it's not the end of the road. She just needs a second opinion (see below).

Step 2: How to prepare for the appointment

Help her build a rock-solid case

Doctors work with evidence. Help her track her symptoms over time – when they started, how often they occur, and how they affect her. Encourage her to write down everything she notices – no matter how small – or share a notebook or app you can both update.

You can also use the Midlife MOT (see Chapter 9) to track key health markers like energy, mood, motivation and libido. Patterns speak louder than feelings – and the more detail she has, the more convincing her case.

Get clear on her goal

What's her objective? It's a simple question, but the answer might not be obvious. Is she seeking a formal diagnosis of perimenopause – that unlocks treatment options like HRT and long-term support? Does she want a referral to a menopause clinic, gynaecologist or mental health expert? Or is she worried it could be something else and wants reassurance?

Having an objective makes the appointment focused and productive. Without one, it's easy to leave feeling frustrated, confused or ignored. If she's unsure, ask what a good result would look like: answers, next steps, or just to be taken seriously?

Note the symptoms, nail the questions

Once she's noted her symptoms and the impact, and decided on a good outcome, a few prepared questions can keep things on track:

- Could these symptoms be perimenopause?
- What treatment options are available?
- Can we talk about HRT – including benefits, risks and types?
- Is there anything else it could be, and are there tests to check?
- What happens next?

She doesn't need to script the entire conversation – just bullet points to stay focused and ensure nothing gets missed.

Offer to be her wingman

Even if she doesn't want you at the appointment with her, the offer counts. If she's on the fence, reassure her you'll only be there to listen, take notes and hold her hand – not to take over or talk for her. She may feel awkward discussing some symptoms with a doctor or in front of you. That's normal. Tell her no one's judging – they just want to understand.

Step 3: How to make the appointment count

Give a last-minute team talk

Whether she's going alone or with you, give her a quick pep talk. Remind her what she feels is real and valid. Remind her to look at her notes, ask her questions, and say what she wants. If nerves are getting the better of her, a simple statement – 'I think I might be in perimenopause, and I'd like to talk about my symptoms' – will get the ball rolling.

Once inside, let her lead and make notes. If she downplays her symptoms, find the right moment to offer your perspective, with sympathetic examples. At the end, remind her of anything she's forgotten to raise.

Use the right words and be specific

Language matters. The right words will paint a clear picture of what she's dealing with. Vague phrases – 'I'm tired' or 'I'm not myself' – are easy to dismiss. GPs hear them all day.

But statements like 'I'm exhausted every day,' 'I keep forgetting things, which makes work impossible,' or 'I haven't slept more than four hours in weeks' are hard to ignore. If she can't find the words, your gentle prompts can help.

Record the conversation, so nothing gets missed

Ask the GP if one of you can record the appointment. It's almost impossible to absorb everything in the moment, especially when emotions are high. Listening back later makes it easier to understand, reflect and plan the next steps with confidence.

Watch how the doctor responds

A good doctor will listen carefully, ask thoughtful questions and explain things clearly. They'll talk through available treatments and other support options.

A dismissive doctor might check the clock, interrupt or try to shut the conversation down. Watch out for phrases like 'It's just stress' or 'That's normal for your age' that signal it's time for a second opinion.

> ### Brush-off bingo: How to tell if it's time for a second opinion
>
> Some doctors are worth their weight in gold. They listen. They understand that menopause can knock her sideways. And they really want to help. If you can get an appointment with a GP who has relevant experience, grab it.
>
> But not every doctor is up to speed. Some are still stuck in the 1950s, tossing out platitudes and antidepressants like confetti at a wedding. So how do you know if she's getting support or being shown the door?
>
> #### Eyes down for brush-off bingo!
>
> If you hear any of the phrases on this board – from 'We all feel low at times!' to 'Try to relax more!' – it's a red flag that her health isn't in the right hands.
>
> Jokes aside, these comments might sound harmless. Well-meaning, even. But they can leave women feeling gaslit, dismissed and completely isolated. So if you hear more than a couple, she needs someone who really understands what she's going through.

BRUSH-OFF BINGO

You're just a bit tired	Have you tried relaxing more?	Everyone's stressed these days	What do you expect at your age?	Your lifestyle is to blame
We all feel a bit down sometimes	Sounds a bit like PMT	Antidepressants will sort you out	Have you tried losing weight?	Stop over-thinking things
Try cutting back on coffee	All women go through this	**BRUSH-OFF BINGO**	It'll settle down eventually	Try getting a bit more sleep
Stop doing too much	Sounds like a bit of anxiety	This is just natural ageing	Try getting some more fresh air	Maybe you need a holiday
Hormones always go up and down	See your friends more often	There's nothing to worry about	All your tests are normal	This is all in your head

Step 4: How to support her after the appointment

Brace for the emotional backlash

If it went well, brilliant – the relief will be huge. But if it didn't, be ready. Many women leave appointments feeling doubted, dismissed or even ridiculed. Don't tell her to calm down or not to worry. That echoes the doctor. Instead listen, validate and support. Remind her she's not wrong – the doctor was. Then help her figure out the next move.

Antidepressants instead of answers?

It's very common for women to be offered antidepressants for perimenopausal symptoms like anxiety, low mood or insomnia[16] – often without hormones getting a mention. Antidepressants can be effective for certain mental health conditions (see Chapter 8), but they won't fix a hormonal imbalance. Unless she has a history of depression or wants to try them, it's worth exploring other options.

Know when to get a second opinion

If the GP lacked knowledge, expertise or sympathy, or she left feeling dismissed or even more confused, ask for another perspective. You have the right to see another doctor. You could also consider private or specialist options – we'll get to these shortly. Whatever you decide, don't wait. Nothing will get better by itself.

Make a plan for what comes next

If it went well, she might leave with an HRT prescription (see Chapter 8), a referral for further tests, or a follow-up appointment. That's progress. If not – or if the advice was vague – make a plan. Whether it's seeing another doctor or seeking clarification, don't let things drift. Even a 'let's wait and see' approach should have a reassessment date – or else you're kicking the can down the road.

When the healthcare system falls short

If multiple GP appointments haven't delivered – or have made things worse – it's time to take a different route.

Private GPs, specialist menopause clinics and reputable online services can offer faster access to professionals who understand what she's going through, and know how to help.

Here's what you need to know about the different options available so she can find the safe, effective and evidence-based care she deserves.

When the NHS isn't enough: Private and online options

Most British people turn to the NHS first, and rightly so. But the UK's public healthcare system is now so overstretched[17] that its focus is increasingly on urgent care and acute illness, not chronic quality-of-life issues like menopause.[18] As we've just covered, GPs often lack the time, training or resources to deal properly with perimenopause, especially when symptoms are vague or unusual.

If she can't get help from her GP, there are other options like private clinics and online providers. Some are excellent. Some aren't. And some simply charge a premium for the exact same treatment she should have got from her GP.

But going private doesn't mean ditching the NHS. Many women use a 'hybrid' approach, starting with a private consultation and prescription, then switching back to the NHS for repeat prescriptions and ongoing care. This can speed things up at the beginning and save money in the long run but only if her NHS doctor agrees to continue her treatment.[19]

Whichever approach she's considering, here's how she can avoid wasting time, money and effort.

Live outside the UK?

Pick up here for everything you need to know about private clinics, online care, and getting the right menopause support when public healthcare isn't part of the picture.

Private healthcare insurance and menopause support

First up, if she has private medical insurance – either personally or through work – check whether menopause care is included. The same goes for employee healthcare schemes.

It's often not. Menopause support is starting to appear in some corporate wellbeing packages, but it's still far from standard. If in doubt, ask HR or the insurance provider directly and get confirmation in writing before booking anything. Even if menopause care is covered, check who she'll actually see. Insurers often refer to consultants rather than menopause specialists, so expertise can vary.

The pros of going private

Private healthcare can be life-changing. The biggest benefits are speed and time. Appointments can happen within days, and you get up to an hour with a menopause specialist. It means avoiding weeks or months of anxious waiting for a ten-minute NHS GP slot in which just one issue can be discussed.[20] Private doctors can also prescribe HRT doses not always available on the NHS.[21]

> ### Medical costs 101
>
> **The price of going private**
>
> Private doesn't always mean better. A fancy website and eye-watering consultation charge doesn't guarantee expertise or empathy. Costs can rise quickly – an initial appointment might set you back £150–£300, with more for prescriptions, blood tests and follow-up reviews.[22]
>
> There are practical issues, too. Depending on where you live, a good clinic might be miles away, and not all have onsite pharmacies. And then some NHS GPs may not accept privately issued test results or treatment plans – hugely frustrating if she wants to move from private to NHS care.[23] That's why it pays to do your homework before splashing the cash.

How to find the right private provider

Going private? Make sure she sees a genuinely qualified menopause specialist. In the UK, look for a General Medical Council-registered doctor or nurse who's completed a recognized menopause qualification. In the US, seek a board-certified OB-GYN or endocrinologist with a similar certification. Once you've identified someone, be prepared with questions about their experience, treatment approach and follow-up care:

- What qualifications do you have in menopause or women's health?
- How many years of experience do you have?
- How many patients do you have?
- What treatments do you offer?
- What are the total costs, including tests, prescriptions and follow-ups?
- How does follow-up care work?

A good provider will welcome these questions. But if the answers are vague, evasive or defensive, walk away. Be especially cautious of woolly phrases like 'hormone balancing' or 'natural reset'. They may sound scientific, but they have no recognized clinical definition or evidence-based backing.

Online menopause clinics: The good, the bad and the dodgy

There's an even faster – and often more affordable – alternative to private clinics: online care.

These services make it easier than ever to speak to a menopause specialist without leaving home. And they're not just digital prescription factories. The best are GP-led, evidence-based and patient-focused.

For many women – especially those juggling work, childcare, low confidence, anxiety and the pressures of midlife – it's a quick, discreet and less daunting option than going to their GP or private clinic. Especially if she's had a bad experience or doesn't want to discuss her health in person.

How online support should work

Online menopause support providers – including Newson Health and Menopause Care in the UK, or Evernow, Alloy and Midi Health in the US – offer fast, flexible access to licensed HRT. Most begin with a symptom questionnaire, followed by a video or phone consultation with a qualified clinician. If appropriate, HRT is prescribed in the format that suits her best, with follow-up check-ins. Blood tests aren't always required – especially for women over 45 – but may be recommended.

Steer clear of the cowboys

The trouble? Not every online clinic has her best interests at heart. While some are run by experienced doctors passionate about women's wellbeing, and follow strict, ethical prescribing protocols, others are little more than slick marketing sites with a prominent 'Pay Now' button designed to separate desperate women from their hard-earned cash.

The main risk with online-only care is misdiagnosis, especially if her symptoms are vague, complex or related to something other than menopause.[24] Without a full history, physical exam or lab work, things can get missed.[25]

Then there can be the hard sell on compounded 'bioidentical' hormones (see Chapter 8) – marketed as natural, personalized and safer than standard HRT. But these products are unregulated, unproven and not recommended by any reputable medical body[26] – including the NHS[27] and the British Menopause Society.[28]

Other red flags include suspect science, miracle claims, no medical credentials, no follow-up, and pressure to buy expensive supplements. Keep in mind that if something sounds too good to be true, it probably is.

When treatment can't wait

If she's found the right provider – whether through the NHS, privately or online – that's a huge step forward. Being taken seriously is half the battle. But understanding what happens next is just as important. It's almost time to talk about treatment options, but first, there's one more medical scenario you might need to know about. One where there's no time to wait.

Not every woman's transition is gradual, and some don't get time to weigh up the options. For women facing surgery, cancer treatment or hormone-suppressing medication, menopause can hit overnight. And when it does, she needs help fast.

Medical menopause – the sudden shutdown

Medical menopause – also known as induced or treatment-induced menopause – happens when certain treatments stop the ovaries from functioning, or they're surgically removed. This causes a sudden and complete drop in oestrogen and other hormones, triggering the same symptoms as natural menopause, but far more abruptly – and often more intensely.

There are no official figures, but it's estimated that up to one in five women may go through a medical menopause.[29] Here are the most common causes:

- **Surgery:** Removal of both ovaries (called bilateral oophorectomy) causes an immediate, permanent menopause.[30] It's sometimes necessary to treat ovarian cancer, reduce the risk of cancer in high-risk women (such as those with the BRCA gene), manage chronic conditions like endometriosis (a painful condition where womb-like tissue grows outside the uterus, often causing severe cramps, inflammation and sometimes infertility), or as a last resort for women experiencing the effects of PMDD (premenstrual dysphoric disorder).[31] And for transgender and non-binary individuals assigned female at birth, the removal of both ovaries as part of gender-affirming surgery causes the same sudden hormone drop. So while not everyone who experiences the menopause identifies as a woman, the symptoms can hit just as hard.

- **Chemotherapy:** Certain cancer treatments can damage the ovaries and impair function, causing temporary or permanent menopause,[32] especially if the drugs are aggressive or treatment is lengthy.
- **Radiation therapy:** Radiation to the pelvic area is used to treat cervical, uterine, ovarian or colorectal cancer. If the ovaries are within the radiation field, they can be damaged or stop working entirely.[33]
- **Hormone-suppressing therapies:** Medications used to treat endometriosis or hormone-sensitive cancers can temporarily shut down ovarian function and cause menopause-like symptoms.[34]

Instant expert

Rachel Mason on supporting her through medical menopause

Rachel Mason is the founder of the wellness supplement brand Our Remedy (ourremedy.co.uk) and a fierce advocate for better hysterectomy and menopause support. She went through a medical menopause at 30 after life-saving cancer surgery and now helps other women, and their partners, feel informed, empowered and less alone.

Be present – physically and emotionally

Whether it's a major surgery or treatment for cancer, this isn't just a medical procedure. It's a huge emotional shift, often involving grief, fear and a loss of identity. She needs practical support and steady reassurance – not distance or silence. Stay close. Knowing she can rely on you, without needing to spell it out, can make the difference between feeling abandoned or safe.

Protect her recovery

If she's had surgery her body needs time to recover and that requires complete rest. If you've got kids or pets, take charge. Do the school runs, the food shop, the errands – in fact, do everything. She'll also need help with the basics: medication reminders, drinks of water, pillows propped, pain relief. If you can't be there in person, set phone alerts to check in.

Respect her grief

Physical scars heal much faster than the emotional ones. Medical menopause often comes with deep, indescribable grief – not just about fertility but identity, control and the future she imagined. You can't fix that, but you can respect it. Don't try to minimize it or brush it off. Just understand that it's real. And don't worry if you're out of your depth – many women find seeing a therapist after medical menopause really helps. You might, too.

Recovery's just the start

This isn't over when she comes home from hospital. She may need long-term HRT, follow-ups, therapy or just someone to help track symptoms. Prove you're in this together. Offer to take notes, chase appointments or read up on what she's been prescribed. Ask questions. Talk to others. The more you understand, the better support you'll be – and the less alone she'll feel.

Let her talk – then really listen

I used to say I was fine when I wasn't. I kept pushing my emotions down, trying not to worry anyone. Many women do the same. What really helps is knowing there's a safe space to talk. So ask gently. Let her know it's OK to open up. Stay close enough for her to feel safe saying what she really needs to say. And when she does? Just listen. That's all you need to do.

Be the difference she deserves

We know there's a lot to take in. But you've done the hard yards. You now know what it takes to help her get the care she needs and deserves. This is what showing up really looks like.

Of all the ways you can support her right now, this might be the biggest. Not by fixing everything. Not by offering answers. But by being there. Helping her weigh up the options. Sitting beside her in the waiting room. Taking notes while she talks. Spotting what the doctor missed. Giving her the confidence to push back when things don't feel right.

In the next chapter, we'll break down what treatment actually looks like – from the pros and cons of HRT to the alternatives and the stuff no one tells you. Because helping her make the right choice doesn't mean making it for her. It means understanding what's out there, asking the smart questions, and standing beside her while she takes back control. That's not just support – that's being the difference.

8

Walking the treatment tightrope
Getting her the support she needs faster

You've both made it this far – through the symptoms, the confusion, the frustration, the appointments. Now it's time to talk treatment. This chapter lifts the lid on the often needlessly confusing world of menopause medication and advice – including hormone replacement therapy – to separate fact from fiction without bias or judgement – so you can help her make an informed choice about her next step.

We'll break down what HRT is, how it works, the pros and cons, and what to do if it's not the right fit, including non-hormonal treatments and alternative therapies. This isn't about pushing pills or playing doctor. It's about helping her feel confident to choose what works for her – in her own time and on her own terms.

In this chapter you'll discover:

- What HRT actually is and how it can help her feel more like herself again
- Why the risks aren't as scary as they sound and the side effects to watch for
- The different types of hormone treatment and how to find the one that fits
- What to expect if she starts HRT and how to support her through the ups and downs
- How testosterone might help bring back her energy, spark and sex drive
- What to do if HRT isn't right for her and why she still has plenty of good options
- The facts about antidepressants, beta blockers and the hormonal coil
- Which alternative therapies may ease her symptoms and help her feel better.

She's seen a GP, had a private appointment, or spoken to an online specialist. For many women now comes the next step: treatment.

That might mean starting HRT – still the most effective option for managing many menopause symptoms.[1] Yet HRT is still shrouded in confusion and controversy. Fear, outdated myths and patchy medical advice have left many women unsure about what it is, how it works, or whether it's dangerous.

Cutting through the HRT confusion

We're going to walk you through what HRT is, how it works, and whether it's right for her. We're also going to cover what happens if she can't take – or doesn't want – HRT, and break down the other treatments that can help. Whether she's ready for HRT, on the fence, or ready to explore other options, this is where you step up again – by knowing the facts, spotting any red flags and supporting her decision. Let's start with the answers to the most common – and most important – HRT questions.

What is hormone replacement therapy?

HRT does exactly what it says on the tin. It replaces the hormones her body is no longer producing as much as it used to – oestrogen (mainly in the form of oestradiol; see below), usually (to be more accurate) progesterone and occasionally testosterone.

Oestrogen is prescribed to ease common symptoms such as hot flushes, night sweats, brain fog and low mood.[2]

If she still has a womb, she'll also need progesterone[3] to stop the lining from thickening, which can increase the risk of cancer.[4] If she's had a hysterectomy (surgical removal of her womb), progesterone isn't needed.

And some women – especially those struggling with libido, energy or motivation – could benefit from testosterone, too,[5] if all other options have been explored. It's not licensed for women in the UK[6] or the US,[7] but it can be prescribed off-label (see below).

Ultimately, there's no one-size-fits-all formula. Her prescription will depend on her symptoms, medical history and personal preferences, including how she wants to take it.

When can she start HRT?

As soon as her symptoms start affecting her quality of life, even if she's still having periods. Some doctors deny women HRT for this reason,[8] but that's outdated thinking. HRT can be started during perimenopause – she doesn't have to wait until she's gone 12 months without a period. In fact, starting HRT during perimenopause may lead to greater health benefits.[9]

What is HRT made from?

Once upon a time, HRT oestrogen only came as oral tablets and was made from the urine of pregnant horses:[10] we're not taking the piss, although someone definitely did.

Thankfully, science and standards have moved on. Today, most of the hormones used in HRT are body-identical (see below) and are made from plant sources like yams and soy.[11]

Oestrogen 101

A quick recap of the hormones that matter

Here's a refresher on the three main types of oestrogen – plus two other key sex hormones – what they do and why they matter.[12]

Oestradiol (E2) – the fertility powerhouse
The strongest and most important form of oestrogen before menopause. Produced by the ovaries, it drives the menstrual cycle and supports mood, memory, bones, skin and heart health. It's the hormone that keeps everything running smoothly – until it doesn't. It's also the main type used in most hormone replacement therapies.[13]

Oestrone (E1) – the post-menopause player
When oestradiol levels fall after menopause, oestrone becomes the dominant oestrogen. It's made in fat tissue and is much weaker, but the body can convert it back to oestradiol if needed, just less efficiently.

Oestriol (E3) – the gentle helper
The weakest of the three types: levels rise during pregnancy but otherwise stay low. It's vital for vaginal and urinary tract health, which is why it's used in local vaginal oestrogen treatments, but not whole-body HRT.

Progesterone – the mood balancer
Produced after ovulation, progesterone helps prepare the womb for pregnancy. It also induces sleep, calms the nervous system and balances mood. After menopause, levels drop sharply, which can trigger symptoms like anxiety, irritability and restlessness.

Testosterone – the missing piece
Women produce testosterone in smaller amounts than men, but still need it to fuel libido, energy, motivation, muscle mass and mental sharpness. Levels gradually decline with age, taking drive and confidence with them.

How is HRT taken?

The most common HRT delivery methods are patches, gels, sprays and tablets.[14] All these deliver hormones into the body, but they work slightly differently. Transdermal options – absorbed through the skin – bypass the liver, which makes them safer for most women,[15] especially those at higher risk of blood clots, stroke, heart disease or gallstones, or those who suffer from migraines (particularly migraine with aura). Tablets must be processed by the liver, which can slightly increase the risk of clots and affect how other medications are broken down[16] – so they're not recommended for women with certain health conditions, including those with obesity or smokers.[17]

- Patches are worn on the skin and changed once or twice a week.
- Gels are rubbed daily onto the skin.
- Sprays are typically used daily on the inner arm.
- Tablets are taken daily by mouth.

Oestrogen is delivered through all these methods. Progesterone, if needed, is usually taken separately, either as an oral tablet, vaginal capsule or hormonal coil (see below). A few combination patches contain both hormones, but these use synthetic progestogen, not body-identical progesterone, so they're falling out of favour despite the convenience.

Just to be clear: progestogen is an umbrella term for all hormones that act like progesterone, including synthetic ones. Progesterone refers specifically to the natural, body-identical hormone.

Less common options include oestrogen implants – small pellets inserted just under the skin of the stomach or bum – which release hormones steadily over many months.[18] These implants are unlicensed in the UK, and because the dose can't be adjusted once they're in, they're typically prescribed by a specialist only when all other forms of HRT haven't worked.[19]

Body-identical, compounded bioidentical or synthetic hormones: What's the difference?

Not all hormones are created equal. These terms sound similar – sometimes deliberately – but they describe very different products with very different risks and results.

Body-identical hormones are chemically identical to those naturally made by the body. They're widely accepted as the gold standard of HRT – produced to strict pharmaceutical standards, approved by regulators, and backed by strong clinical evidence.[20] A GP or qualified clinician can prescribe them in standardized doses via tablets, gels, sprays or patches.

Compounded bioidentical hormones, on the other hand, are custom-mixed by private pharmacies outside the regulatory framework.[21] Often based on saliva or blood tests, they're sold as creams, lozenges or under-the-tongue drops, usually via private clinics or online. Because they're unregulated, there's no guarantee of quality, consistency or safety. Doses can vary from batch to batch, there's no solid evidence they work better than regulated HRT, and they may carry greater risks. That's why they're not recommended by any major medical organization – and best avoided altogether.[22]

Synthetic hormones were common in older types of HRT and are still used in some products today – typically synthetic progestogens in certain combined tablets and patches.[23] These hormones are structurally different from those found in the body and may carry a slightly different risk profile – especially for breast cancer and blood clots – depending on the type, dose and delivery method.

When does HRT start working?

Some symptoms ease within a few days or weeks, especially hot flushes, disrupted sleep and mood swings.[24] Others, like brain fog or low libido, may take a little longer, sometimes several months.[25] If things don't settle – or her symptoms change – it's not a failure. It usually just means the type, dose or delivery method needs adjusting. That's why follow-up appointments matter – to review and adjust her treatment if needed.

How long can she stay on HRT?

A common misconception is that HRT should be taken only for a set time. But there's no rule that says she has to stop. The latest guidance from the British Medical Society is clear: she can stay on HRT for as long as the benefits outweigh the risks.[26] For some women, that means taking it indefinitely. Others may choose to stop after a few years. It's a decision to revisit regularly with her doctor.

Vaginal hormones 101

Rapid relief from problems 'down there'

Vaginal hormones can be prescribed alongside – or instead of – standard HRT. They target local symptoms like dryness, itching, pain during sex, or general discomfort around the vulva and vagina.[27] Unlike other forms of HRT, they aren't absorbed into the bloodstream in significant amounts, so aren't classed as systemic HRT, and they don't increase the risk of breast cancer or blood clots.

They come as creams or gels (applied inside the vagina using an applicator), small pessaries (inserted like a tiny tablet), or a soft ring that slowly releases oestrogen over time. Most products are used daily for a few weeks, then a couple of times a week to maintain results.

They're safe for most women to use long term, even after they have stopped other forms of HRT, and for many, they can be a genuine game changer: easing pain, restoring comfort and reigniting a sex life they thought was gone for good.

Does she need testosterone?

You might think of testosterone as the hormone that makes you hairy and horny – and you'd be right. But women produce it, too, just in much smaller amounts – roughly 7–10 percent of the level found in men.[28]

For most women on HRT, oestrogen does the heavy lifting, but sometimes, it's not quite enough. That's where testosterone may help.[29]

As we covered in Chapter 4, men's testosterone begins to drop steadily from their thirties – by around 1–2 percent a year.[30] For women, the decline starts earlier – from their twenties[31] – and by menopause, their levels may be down to a quarter (or less) or less of their youthful peak.[32]

For some women, that decline matters. Hypoactive sexual desire disorder (HSDD) is a persistent or recurrent lack of sexual thoughts, fantasies or desire that causes significant distress or relationship difficulties,[33] and testosterone therapy can help.[34]

But it's not just about sex drive. Testosterone also plays a role in energy, motivation, mood and more.[35] So topping up low levels can make a meaningful difference. The catch? It's not licensed for women in the UK[36] or the US.[37] It can be prescribed off-label – usually by a menopause specialist,[38] and typically only when other options haven't worked.[39] Many women describe it as life-changing, especially for mood and libido.[40] But it's not for everyone, and it's not a magic bullet. Like all HRT, it's about finding what works for her.

> **It's never too late for HRT!**
>
> Some doctors still claim it's not worth starting HRT after 60. That's wrong.[41] There's no age limit – it just needs the right dose, delivery and oversight. HRT can still ease symptoms, strengthen bones and improve quality of life, even years after menopause.

The case for HRT

HRT isn't just about easing symptoms – it's about helping her feel like herself again. And for many women, the changes come quickly.

According to research from Newson Health,[42] around nine in ten women report relief from hot flushes and night sweats within weeks of starting HRT. Sleep improves for 35 percent, concentration sharpens for 34 percent, and energy returns for 32 percent. Mood lifts as anxiety eases. Libido bounces back, too, as vaginal dryness, itching or discomfort often disappear. And while every woman's experience is different, many say the lift in mental load – and the return of emotional resilience and control – is just as powerful as the physical relief.

The long-term benefits are equally compelling. Starting HRT before 60 significantly reduces the risk of cardiovascular disease and all-cause mortality.[43] It's also linked to improved cognitive function and a lower risk of dementia,[44] along with up to a 30 percent reduction in osteoporosis-related fractures.[45]

Tracking symptoms over time helps her get the most from treatment. A symptom diary shows what's getting better, what still needs work, and whether a tweak in dose or delivery might help. The Midlife MOT in Chapter 9 is a simple weekly check-in that helps her keep track of how she's feeling – physically, mentally and emotionally – and what's worth raising at her next appointment.

The big benefits of HRT

HRT isn't just about taking the edge off. For many women restoring hormonal balance brings back what's been missing and helps them feel like themselves again. Here are the most common, evidence-backed improvements reported after starting treatment.

Short-term benefits[46]

Often noticeable within days or weeks, though some may take longer to improve:

- Relief from hot flushes and night sweats
- Better sleep – both quality and duration
- Improved mood and reduced anxiety
- Sharper thinking and less brain fog
- More energy and motivation
- Reduced vaginal dryness and discomfort, and renewed sex drive (especially with vaginal oestrogen)

Long-term benefits

Develop over months and years:

- Stronger bones and reduced risk of osteoporosis-related fractures[47]
- Improved heart health, especially when started before age 60 or within ten years of menopause[48]
- Possible protection against cognitive decline and dementia (evidence strongest with early use and body-identical hormones)[49]
- Reduced risk of diabetes,[50] bowel cancer,[51] auto-immune disease[52] and clinical depression[53]

What are the risks of HRT?

If there's one thing most people think they know about HRT, it's this: it increases the risk of breast cancer.

This claim has circulated for decades, but the dangers have often been exaggerated, misreported or misunderstood. That's led to fear, confusion and hesitation – not just among women but among doctors, too.[54] The truth is more balanced.[55] Yes, there are risks. But they're much smaller than many people realize, and for most women in good health, the benefits greatly exceed them.[56]

HRT and breast cancer: The truth behind the headlines

In 2002, a Women's Health Initiative (WHI) study made global headlines by reporting an increased risk of breast cancer, stroke and heart disease in women taking HRT. Almost overnight, millions of women stopped treatment, and many doctors became reluctant to prescribe it.[57] Fear around HRT was rampant.

But what wasn't highlighted at the time was that the WHI study had serious flaws.[58] Most of the women studied were in their sixties and seventies – well past menopause – and many had existing health issues, including obesity, high blood pressure and a history of smoking.[59] They were also given types of synthetic hormones that are rarely prescribed today.[60]

More recent evidence shows that starting HRT around the time menopause symptoms begin – and using today's regulated, body-identical hormones – offers significantly more benefits than risks.[61] Yet many women – and many doctors – are still influenced[62] by those alarming headlines, even though the actual risk of cancer or disease linked to HRT is very small compared to lifestyle risks such as obesity, alcohol or inactivity (see below).

We're not pushing HRT as the right choice for every woman. We simply want you, and her, to have the full picture – based on the latest evidence, not outdated fears – so she can make the right choice for her body, her symptoms and her long-term health.

How do HRT risks compare to other factors?

Yes, there is a slightly higher risk of breast cancer with some types of HRT, particularly when used long term, and especially when using synthetic progestogens.[63] But these are increasingly being phased out in favour of body-identical progesterone, which carries a lower risk profile.

So how big is the risk? Combined HRT (oestrogen plus synthetic progestogen) is associated with around one to two extra cases of breast cancer per 1,000 women per year.[64] That risk begins to decline once treatment stops.

There is also a small risk of blood clots and stroke, mainly in older women taking oral oestrogen and those taking a synthetic progestogen.[65]

For younger, healthy women using transdermal options (patches, gels or sprays), the risk is extremely low, because these methods bypass the liver and don't appear to affect clotting in the same way.[66]

For some perspective, those risks are significantly lower than these common lifestyle factors:

- **Obesity** more than doubles the risk of postmenopausal breast cancer.[67]
- One **alcoholic drink** a day raises breast cancer risk by up to 10 percent, while two or three increases it to 20 percent.[68]
- **Smoking** is linked to a 10–20 percent higher risk of breast cancer depending on smoking duration and quantity.[69]
- A **sedentary lifestyle** is estimated to raise breast cancer risk by up to 15.5 percent.[70]

Why we panic about HRT, but not the pill or Viagra

For women with a history of breast cancer, HRT is usually off the table – but not always.[71] It depends on the type of cancer, whether it was oestrogen-receptor positive or triple-negative (which doesn't respond to hormones). Either way, it's a decision that needs to involve both an oncologist and a menopause specialist.

It's also worth knowing that the hormone doses used in modern HRT are relatively low compared to the combined oral contraceptive pill,[72] which millions of women take for years without facing anywhere near the same level of fear or controversy. And the hormones used in the pill are almost always synthetic, not body-identical.[73]

Final thought: Viagra is taken by millions of men worldwide without anyone batting an eyelid (they're probably too busy staring at something else), despite it carrying a higher immediate risk of many health conditions, including low blood pressure, vision changes, and, in rare cases, a heart attack or stroke.[74] And that risk is willingly accepted for just 15 minutes of feeling like your old self. HRT offers much more and lasts far longer.

> ### The fruit and herb that hurt HRT
>
> Oral HRT can be affected by certain foods and supplements – grapefruit can raise hormone levels,[75] while St John's wort can lower them.[76] These don't affect patches, gels or sprays, which bypass the liver.[77] Always check the labels on medications and supplements for possible side effects.

Still confused? Let's bust the biggest HRT myths

Despite everything we now know, many myths still muddy the waters. Here's the truth behind seven of the most common HRT misunderstandings.

Myth 1: HRT increases the risk of breast cancer

The risk is small and depends on the type, dose and how long it's taken. For most healthy women under 60, the benefits far outweigh the risks – especially with body-identical hormones and transdermal options.[78]

Myth 2: HRT is only for hot flushes or serious symptoms

It can also help with mood, memory, sex drive, sleep, joint pain and more.[79] HRT is for anyone whose quality of life is being affected.

Myth 3: You need a blood test to get HRT

You don't. Hormone levels fluctuate constantly during perimenopause so symptoms are often more reliable than lab results. The caveat? If she's under 45,[80] blood tests may be done, in part to rule out other concerns.

Myth 4: You can't start HRT if you're still having periods

Wrong. HRT can be most effective when started during perimenopause, when hormones swing wildly and symptoms often hit hardest.[81]

Myth 5: HRT only masks menopause symptoms

It replaces hormones the body has stopped making. For many women, that means better daily wellbeing and better health in the long run.[82]

Myth 6: Natural supplements are safer

Many so-called 'natural' remedies are unproven and unregulated.[83] Regulated, body-identical HRT is clinically tested, safe and effective, and backed by decades of research.

Myth 7: You can't take HRT for ever / You must take HRT for life

There's no fixed limit. She can stay on HRT for as long as the benefits outweigh the risks[84] – as long as she's having regular reviews. Some women stay on it long term; others choose to stop when their symptoms settle or they simply don't want it anymore.

Ozempic 101

The truth about weight-loss jabs and HRT

Weight-loss injections promise fast and effortless results, but what do they mean for midlife women already navigating hormonal upheaval?

For decades, people dreamed of a wonder drug that could melt away stubborn fat in weeks. No gym. No diet. No effort. Then it arrived: injectable medications that suppress appetite, slow digestion and trigger rapid weight loss. But as with any so-called miracle fix, be careful what you wish for, especially if you're a woman in midlife.

Ozempic and Wegovy (brand names for semaglutide) and Mounjaro (tirzepatide) belong to a class of drugs called GLP-1 receptor agonists.[85] They mimic a gut hormone that regulates hunger, blood sugar and digestion, helping you feel fuller for longer – so you eat less without even trying.

From medical miracle to short-cut craze

Originally developed to treat type-2 diabetes, these drugs are now licensed in the UK for people with obesity (BMI 30+) or a BMI of 27+ with related health issues like high blood pressure or cholesterol. For those patients, the benefits can be life-changing – even life-saving.

But their dramatic effects have fuelled demand beyond those guidelines. Private clinics, online services and even social media influencers now sell them as a short cut to slimness, especially to women battling perimenopausal weight gain.

Yet these drugs pose two big problems for women in midlife.

First: you don't just lose fat. Studies show these drugs can significantly reduce muscle mass and bone density[86] – two things that are already shrinking during perimenopause. That smaller number on the scale could come at a greater cost to long-term strength, resilience and health.

Second: these drugs slow down how quickly food – and medications – moves through the gut. This can affect how oral HRT is absorbed: progesterone, in particular, may not be taken up properly, reducing the protection it offers the womb lining. (It's worth adding that they may also interfere with how well the contraceptive pill works, so other methods of birth control are advised.)

That's why the British Menopause Society (BMS) recommends women on GLP-1 drugs switch to non-oral options: transdermal oestrogen and a progesterone-releasing IUD, like Mirena.[87]

Potent – but not without problems

Ozempic isn't actually licensed for weight loss in the UK – only for treating type-2 diabetes. Wegovy and Mounjaro are the only GLP-1 jabs approved for weight management, and only for people with clinical need under proper medical supervision.[88]

Some private clinics will prescribe Ozempic off-label, which is technically legal but discouraged by both the BMS[89] and the Medicines and Healthcare products Regulatory Agency.[90]

These are powerful drugs, and yes, they can be transformative. But used without the right diagnosis, monitoring and support, they may do more harm than good. If your partner is considering them, make sure she talks to a qualified health professional first.

HRT side effects and the warning signs

Starting HRT can set her on course for greater health and happiness, but it isn't always plain sailing at first. Many women feel better within days or weeks, but some experience mild side effects as their body adjusts to the new hormone levels. These are usually nothing to worry about, but it's crucial to know what's normal at the start and what's not.

Normal side effects

During the first 6–12 weeks, it's common to experience:[91]

- Light vaginal bleeding or spotting
- Headaches
- Breast tenderness
- Bloating
- Nausea
- Mood swings or irritability.

These usually settle as her body finds its new balance. But if symptoms persist or worsen, she should speak to her doctor. It doesn't mean HRT isn't working – just that the dose or delivery might need tweaking.

What's not normal and needs investigation

Certain side effects may signal a bigger issue and should never be ignored. If she experiences any of the following, there's no need to panic but she should speak to a healthcare professional as soon as possible:[92]

- Heavy or unexpected vaginal bleeding
- Severe or persistent headaches
- Calf pain or swelling (a possible sign of a blood clot)
- Chest pain or shortness of breath
- Vision changes
- New or worsening depression or anxiety
- Skin irritation from patches that doesn't improve
- Any symptom that feels extreme or out of the ordinary.

Finding the right fit

It can take time to get the combination just right. Most issues can be resolved by adjusting the type, dose or delivery of HRT. That might mean switching from a tablet to a patch, trying a different progesterone, or increasing or lowering the oestrogen dose.

This isn't failure – it's fine-tuning.

And that's why regular check-ins are so important, especially in the early months. A good menopause specialist will review how she's feeling, track what's changing, and help tweak her treatment to suit her body and her needs.

Over time, HRT should be reviewed once a year to check what's working, what's not, and whether her needs have changed.[93] It's a chance to reflect on what's improved, what still needs attention, and how treatment can evolve with her.

Instant expert

Kate Muir on what every woman needs to know about HRT

Kate Muir is a journalist, campaigner and author of Everything You Need to Know about the Menopause (But Were Too Afraid to Ask).[94]

She wrote and produced Sex, Myths and the Menopause *with Davina McCall, the groundbreaking Channel 4 documentary that changed the conversation about HRT and helped drive a million more women towards treatment (katemuir.co.uk).*

Fear is still holding women back

The myth that HRT causes breast cancer came from one flawed study back in 2002. It used outdated, synthetic hormones on older women with health risks, and it scared a generation off HRT. The truth? The newer, body-identical hormones used today are considerably safer, and for most women the benefits far outweigh the small risks. But the fear lingers, and too many women are still suffering.

Most doctors aren't up to speed

The scientific understanding of menopause has moved on dramatically, but the medical system hasn't caught up. There's a whole new wave of menopause science, and a growing movement of doctors pushing for change. But until things improve, women are often left to figure it out themselves – learning to recognize their symptoms and push for the right treatment when no one else will.

HRT revealed what was really going on

When I went through menopause, I wasn't having hot flushes – I was having memory lapses and heart palpitations. I thought I had early-onset Alzheimer's. Within a week of starting HRT, my memory came back. So many symptoms – from anxiety to joint pain – are hormonal. But many women don't know, and doctors don't ask.

Getting the right treatment takes time

She might not get the right dose or combination straight away. It took me five years to get mine right – I had to switch forms and figure out what worked for my body. Everyone absorbs oestrogen differently. On the average dose of two pumps a day, I still get the odd hot flush. On three, I don't – that's my dose, discovered through trial and error and signed off by my NHS GP. Body-identical progesterone can also make a huge difference. It's never one-size-fits-all. But once she finds what works, it can be life-changing. Don't give up.

> **Beware the menopause money machine**
>
> The menopause industry is now worth billions, but not all of it helps women. From fancy supplements to dodgy diagnostics and 'biohacking' clinics, there's a lot of noise. Many people are monetizing fear. HRT is cheap, effective, evidence-based and widely available – it costs about £8 ($11) a month on the NHS, while some over-the-counter 'menopause vitamins' cost £30. Women don't need expensive fixes – they need accurate information and access to proper care.
>
> **This is about power, not pills**
>
> HRT isn't about eternal youth – it's about strength, energy and living well for longer. It protects her brain, bones and heart. It can give her back her career, her confidence, her relationship – her life. I've seen it. I've lived it. And I'll keep shouting about it until every woman knows what's possible.

Why she might say no to HRT

Not every woman can take – or wants – HRT. Whatever the reason, it's her body and her choice – so give her the support she deserves whatever she decides.

When it's not advised

Body-identical HRT might not be suitable if she has:[95]

- had hormone-sensitive cancer (like breast or womb cancer)
- unexplained vaginal bleeding
- severe side effects from HRT in the past.

When she chooses not to

Even if it's safe, she might still say no – and that's her call. Common reasons include:[96]

- Worries about side effects or long-term risks
- A preference for natural or non-medical approaches
- Personal or cultural beliefs about hormones
- Previous bad experiences with doctors or medication
- Mild symptoms she feels she can manage without treatment.

> ### How shame keeps women suffering in silence
> It's not just fear of side effects that puts women off HRT. More than one in three report feeling shame or stigma around their menopause symptoms.[97] That emotional weight can make a woman reluctant to seek help or consider HRT, especially if she sees it as 'cheating' or a 'cop out', or fears being judged for needing medical support during a 'natural' life stage. It's a bit like refusing pain relief during childbirth. Sounds mad, right? Why turn down something that could help so much? Don't underestimate the social expectations, cultural baggage and peer pressure women face. It's enough to make many suffer in silence rather than seek the relief they deserve.

When HRT isn't right for her

When HRT isn't suitable – or she doesn't want it – she's not out of options. There are other evidence-based treatments that can ease symptoms and improve quality of life, with or without hormones. Some of these were originally developed for other conditions but can help with hot flushes, night sweats or low mood. Others support better sleep, mental health and day-to-day wellbeing. Here's what she might be offered.

Antidepressants

Antidepressants aren't usually the first choice for menopause symptom relief but some can help reduce the frequency and intensity of hot flushes and night sweats.[98]

The most commonly prescribed are SSRIs (selective serotonin reuptake inhibitors) or SNRIs (serotonin-norepinephrine reuptake inhibitors), such as venlafaxine, commonly prescribed as Efexor XL (Effexor in the US), or fluoxetine, better known as Prozac.

They don't offer instant relief – it usually takes a few weeks to feel any benefit – and some women may feel worse before they feel better.[99]

They can also come with side effects such as nausea, dizziness, low libido or sleep disturbances.[100] And if her symptoms are mainly hormonal, HRT is likely to be more effective.

If she's really struggling with anxiety, low mood or panic attacks, antidepressants may be part of the solution – with or without HRT. It's about finding the right fit for her symptoms and her mental health needs.

Beta blockers

Beta blockers reduce the physical symptoms of anxiety – like a racing heart, shaking or palpitations – by blocking the effects of adrenaline on the heart and blood vessels.[101] Unlike antidepressants, which take time to work, beta blockers offer fast-acting relief in high-stress moments. And while they don't treat the underlying cause, they can be a useful short-term tool while exploring longer-term solutions like HRT, therapy or lifestyle changes.

Contraceptive pill

The combined oral contraceptive pill is sometimes offered by doctors as a way to manage symptoms like irregular bleeding or mood swings. The problem? It contains synthetic hormones at much higher doses than HRT, and it masks what's really going on hormonally.[102] Some pills also increase the risk of blood clots and may not be suitable for women over 35, especially those who are obese, smoke or have other risk factors.[103]

Hormonal coil

A hormonal coil is an IUD (intrauterine device) that delivers a steady, low dose of a synthetic progestogen (levonorgestrel) directly into the womb. Of the available options, Mirena is the best studied and most widely recommended for the progestogen component of HRT.[104]

These devices are used for contraception, but are also very effective at protecting the womb lining when used alongside oestrogen as part of HRT.[105] The coil is commonly offered to women who have very heavy, prolonged or painful periods, as it can reduce menstrual bleeding and in some cases stop it altogether.[106] Although the hormone is released into the womb, it still enters the bloodstream and can cause systemic side effects in some women. That said, the coil remains a convenient, low-maintenance option that can stay in place for up to five years,[107] making it a practical choice for women who want contraception, HRT or both.

Clonidine

Clonidine is a blood pressure medication that can help reduce hot flushes and night sweats by affecting the brain's temperature regulation system.[108] It's not as effective as HRT, and side effects – dry mouth, dizziness, constipation and low blood pressure – are common.[109]

Gabapentin

Gabapentin is prescribed for epilepsy or nerve pain, but may reduce the intensity of sweating and flushes, particularly at night.[110] It is a controlled drug, meaning it's legally restricted due to the risk of addiction and misuse, and it can cause side effects including dizziness and drowsiness.[111] It's generally only prescribed off-label if other options haven't worked.[112]

Cognitive behavioural therapy (CBT)

CBT is a type of talking therapy that helps people change unhelpful patterns of thinking or behaviour. It's been adapted specifically for menopause and is recommended by NICE for managing low mood, anxiety and sleep problems as well as how symptoms are perceived.[113]

While it doesn't treat hormonal changes directly, CBT can improve how she copes with them, reducing stress, improving resilience and boosting quality of life.

It's particularly useful for women who can't take HRT, or who still feel overwhelmed despite taking it. CBT is available on the NHS in some areas, or privately through a qualified therapist. Online and group options are also available.

Alternative therapies

These alternative and complementary therapies are popular among women looking for natural options, and some find them helpful. However, the evidence for their effectiveness is mixed.

Acupuncture may help reduce hot flushes and improve sleep in some women, though results vary and benefits often depend on the practitioner's experience.[114] It's generally considered safe, but effects are usually mild and gradual.

Yoga can support physical and mental wellbeing, especially when it includes breathing, relaxation and mindfulness. It won't treat hormonal changes directly, but can ease stress, improve sleep and boost energy and mood[115] – all of which matter during menopause.

Herbal remedies such as black cohosh, red clover and St John's wort are widely marketed for menopause symptoms.[116] Some contain phytoestrogens – plant compounds that mimic oestrogen – but their effects are weaker and less consistent than HRT. Some also interact with other medications or come with health risks.[117] That's why she should speak to a pharmacist or doctor before trying anything new. Remember, the best outcomes are from a tailored approach – one that reflects her symptoms, her situation and her say.

Instant expert

Dr Philippa Kaye on why a personalized approach matters

Dr Philippa Kaye is a GP, author[118] and broadcaster specializing in women's health (drphilippakaye.com). She believes menopause care should be based on the individual – not a checklist or blood test – and that good medicine means helping every woman find the right support for her needs.

The person in front of me matters most

There's no one way to manage menopause. No two women will have the same experience, and no two women will need exactly the same treatment. My first job is always to listen. What are her symptoms? How is it affecting her life? What does she want from treatment? Good care starts with treating the individual, not ticking boxes or following a flowchart.

Symptoms are more important than blood tests

One of the biggest misunderstandings in menopause care is the idea that you need to diagnose it with a blood test. The menopause is defined as the last menstrual period – once you haven't bled for a year, you have been through the menopause. The perimenopause is the period of time before the menopause where you may have symptoms. If you are over 45 years old, blood tests are not needed to diagnose the perimenopause. We can go on symptoms alone because hormone levels bounce around all over the place during perimenopause. A test might come back 'normal' even if a woman is clearly struggling. That's why we base diagnosis on symptoms, history and the overall picture – not just on lab results. Under the age of 45, blood tests are needed, especially to exclude other causes.

HRT should be an informed choice, not an automatic prescription

HRT can be life-changing for many women, but it isn't the right choice for everyone. My role is to explain the benefits and the risks, in the context of that woman's health, goals and life stage. Some women will want HRT straight away. Others may want to try non-hormonal treatments or other approaches first. Both are valid. My job isn't to persuade her one way or the other – it's to make sure she has the information she needs to make the decision that feels right for her.

Mental health symptoms deserve real attention

Mood swings, anxiety, low resilience, feeling overwhelmed – these are all very real symptoms of perimenopause. And they can be devastating. I see so many women who have been told they're simply depressed or stressed, without anyone looking at the hormonal changes driving those feelings. Treating mood alone without addressing the hormonal cause means women often don't get the full help they need. We have to join the dots between mind and body.

Good menopause care is about options, not ultimatums

There are many ways to manage menopause. HRT is one tool, but it's not the only one. CBT can help. Exercise and diet can make a difference. Non-hormonal medications can ease some symptoms. Sometimes it's a combination of approaches that works best. What matters most is that women feel they have choices – real, informed, personalized choices – not that they're being pushed down a path that doesn't fit them. Good care respects those choices and supports women to find their way through.

> ### She's reclaiming her power – thanks to you
>
> Whichever path she chooses – HRT, non-hormonal options, both or neither – the fact that you're by her side means you've already done more than most men ever do. You leaned in, you listened, and you helped her tune out the fear and reclaim her power, so she can figure out what works for her body and her life. That matters. It changes everything.
>
> And speaking of power – that's the theme of the final section of this book. You've got the knowledge. You've cracked the communication. Now it's time to take back control of your lives. Sleep better. Stress less. Eat smarter. Move more. Because this isn't just about surviving – it's about thriving. The life you imagined? It starts now. Healthier. Happier. Stronger. Together.

Part 3
POWER

Part 3
POWER

9

Stress less and sleep deep
Rapidly recharge both body and mind

Kicking off the Power section of the book, this chapter is packed with smart, simple, real-world advice to help you both not just survive perimenopause but also thrive through it. And the best part? There's far more in your control than you might think. We'll reveal the quick and easy ways to manage stress and improve sleep. Then everything else gets easier. In Chapters 10 and 11, we'll cover food and exercise, and how some quick wins can transform how you both look and feel – fast.

It's time to cut through the noise and focus on what actually works – backed by experts, grounded in science and proven in real life. And this doesn't mean overhauling your entire lives. Just a few small steps in the right direction will make a massive difference to her health and happiness – and yours, too.

In this chapter you'll discover:

- Why now is the perfect time to take action – for her health and yours
- How hormonal and lifestyle changes affect the body, and what you can do about it
- The four key lifestyle pillars that support better health, energy and resilience
- How to use the Midlife MOT to track your progress and keep each other motivated
- Why you don't need to fix everything at once, and how to start where it matters most
- Why stress and sleep are the foundations of feeling better fast
- How to take control of stress and stay calm under pressure, even when life's kicking off
- How to sort your sleep so you stop waking up shattered and start running on full power.

Welcome to the Power section of the book. Been a bit of a ride getting here, huh?

Don't worry if you feel overwhelmed. That's normal. In fact, if you're not even slightly anxious, you've almost certainly underestimated the gravity of the situation you're now in. Maybe go back and read Chapter 2 again – this time without the football on in the background.

All the talk about signs and symptoms, treatment pros and cons, and dealing with doctors is a lot to get your head around. Especially if you didn't even know what perimenopause was before you picked up (or were handed) this book.

Turning panic into power

But now is your chance to shine. No cape or tights required – just a willingness to show up as the everyday hero she needs.

And it couldn't have come at a better time. Why? Because she's probably never felt this awkward and uncomfortable in her own skin, or this unhappy with how her body looks, feels and functions. It can shatter her confidence and make her feel as though her life's spinning out of control.

You're about to be armed with everything you need to help her take back control of her health and happiness – and your own, too.

A stranger in her own body

Before you can help her move forward, you need to understand what's holding her back. Perimenopause doesn't just change how a woman feels – it can also change how she looks. And not in ways she expected or wanted.

These physical changes can be sudden and dramatic: the average woman gains 1.5kg (3.3lb) per year during perimenopause,[1] and puts on a total of 10kg – more than one and a half stone – by the time she reaches menopause (see 'What is a "healthy" weight?' below).[2]

Weight gain alone is bad enough. But it's where that weight goes that's the real problem.

Hormones, muffin tops and love handles

Hormones influence how and where we store fat. As oestrogen falls, her body starts redirecting it to her tummy – not to her hips, thighs, bum or boobs, where it used to go.[3] Men in lab coats call it 'visceral fat accumulation' or 'abdominal adiposity'. Men with a death wish call it 'menopause belly' or 'meno belly'. Our advice? Best not to say any of those out loud. In fact, let's just pretend we never mentioned it.

What's harder to carry than the extra weight is how it makes her feel. Chances are, she won't come right out and tell you how unhappy she is with her body – maybe out of confusion or embarrassment, or because she doesn't have the words yet. Still, there will be signs. A mountain of clothes destined for the charity shop. A tearful meltdown before a night out because 'nothing fucking fits'. Or something more subtle – like a sudden obsession with true crime podcasts about women who murder their husbands.

Who's the man in the mirror?

But let's be honest – it's not just her body that's changing size and shape. When you got out of the shower this morning and caught sight of your reflection, how did you feel?

Man boobs, dad bod and beer belly – they're all funny phrases. But they're no laughing matter. They stop clothes fitting. They make you feel self-conscious out of them. And – no sugarcoating this – they can leave you feeling pretty shitty about yourself.[4]

And what about your mood and motivation?[5] More of us than ever are struggling with energy and drive,[6] while our bellies win the war against our elasticated waistbands.[7]

A trickle versus a tsunami

The big difference is that for us blokes, these changes don't happen overnight. They're the result of thousands of small decisions – those 'I'll start on Monday' missed gym sessions really do add up – like a slow trickle of water wearing down rock over many years.

But for women, plummeting oestrogen levels mean these changes come like a tsunami – fast, overwhelming, and devastating to both body and mind.

While your changes aren't so sudden, they're just as problematic. Being overweight, overtired and overstressed affects your body composition (more belly fat, less muscle), and increases your risk of obesity, heart disease and cancer.[8] It also lowers your testosterone,[9] which – as we covered in Chapter 4 – already drops by about 1–2 percent per year from your thirties. A faster fall can further hit your mood, motivation and mojo.[10]

Body fat 101

What is a 'healthy' weight?

There's no one magic number. What's healthy for you depends on your age, gender, height, body shape, activity levels and more. But there are sensible guidelines worth knowing – not to obsess over, but to help you stay on top of your health.

As you get older and hormone levels shift, it's normal to see changes in muscle, bone and body fat. But if your weight's creeping up – especially around your middle – it can be an early warning sign for a whole range of health issues.[11]

The key to maintaining a healthy weight is tracking the metrics that actually matter. Some methods are useful. Others are a waste of time. Here's what you need to know.

Bathroom scales

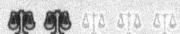

What? Found in most bathrooms and gyms, these scales are the simplest and quickest option, but only measure total body weight – without distinguishing between muscle mass (good), excess fat mass (bad) or water retention (variable).
How? Strip off, step on and note the number.
Useful? Not really. During perimenopause hormonal changes can cause wild weight fluctuations that can be misleading. And the lack of clarity between lean (muscle and bone) mass and fat mass gives a blurry picture of overall health for both women and men.

Smart scales

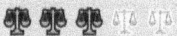

What? Smart scales use a mild electrical pulse to estimate body fat percentage, muscle mass and other metrics – along with total weight – though accuracy can vary.
How? Stand still on the scales in your birthday suit. The readings will appear on the digital display or sync to an app.

Useful? More helpful than simple scales because they track fat and muscle changes – but water retention can skew the data.

Body mass index (BMI)

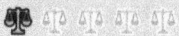

What? Still widely used in medicine, BMI calculates weight relative to height, but it doesn't account for muscle mass, fat percentage, or where fat is stored.
How? Get a calculator. Take your weight in kilograms and divide it by your height in metres squared (kg/m²). A BMI between 18.5 and 24.9 is considered healthy.
Useful? Nope. BMI won't flag up body composition changes in perimenopause and often misclassifies muscular men as overweight.

Waist-to-height ratio

⚖️ ⚖️ ⚖️ ⚖️ ⚖️

What? It measures how much fat is stored around your belly in proportion to your height, and it's a strong predictor of long-term health.
How? Measure your waist at its narrowest then divide the number by your height in centimetres. Aim for a score below 0.5.
Useful? Very – it's arguably the best method for tracking weight-related health risks because belly fat is a major warning sign for conditions like heart disease and type-2 diabetes.

Waist-to-hip ratio

⚖️ ⚖️ ⚖️ ⚖️ ⚖️

What? It compares waist size to hip size to assess where fat is distributed and what that means for your health.
How? Measure your waist at its narrowest point and your hips at their widest, then divide the waist measurement by the hip measurement. A healthy ratio is under 0.85 for women and 0.9 for men.
Useful? Yes. In women, it reflects the hormonal shift from a pear-shaped to an apple-shaped body, which comes with greater health risks. In men, it highlights belly weight gain and the problems that come with it.

Weighing up the options

As we explained in Chapters 4 (you) and 8 (her), hormone replacement therapy can ease or erase some of the mental and physical health issues that arise in midlife.

But HRT isn't the only answer. Whether or not it's an option either of you wants to explore, some simple tweaks to your daily routine can have a profound impact on how you look, feel and perform. For some women, lifestyle changes can take certain perimenopause symptoms from intolerable to manageable, or maybe even eradicate some completely.[12] That's obviously great news for her. But it's very good news for you, too.

Why? Because almost all the smart, simple, science-backed advice that follows – how to stress less to stay sane, sleep better to boost energy, eat well to lose weight, and exercise more to feel better – applies just as much to you as to her.

The four pillars of a healthy and happy life

This chapter – and the next couple – focus on the four pillars that underpin better health, energy and vitality: stress, sleep, nutrition and exercise.

Rather than isolated islands, these four pillars are actually four interconnected circles, so improving one area has a positive knock-on effect on the others. For instance, a bit more exercise reduces stress, which improves sleep, which makes eating well easier – which boosts your energy and motivation to exercise again.[13] And round it goes.

On the flip side, that virtuous cycle can quickly turn vicious: a sedentary lifestyle raises stress, wrecks sleep, and leads to poor food choices – making even the thought of exercise exhausting.[14]

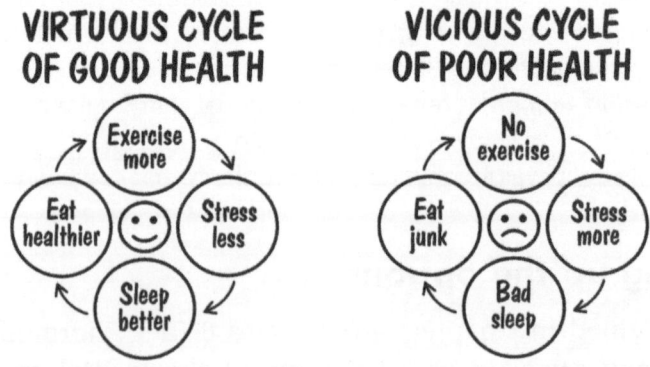

Small steps, big wins

Luckily, it's surprisingly easy to get the virtuous cycle turning. All you need to do is pick one lifestyle pillar to start with – stress, sleep, food or fitness – and put our expert advice into action.

That's right. You don't have to change everything all at once. The smartest approach? Start small, stay specific, and take it one step at a time.[15]

Take stock before you start

Before you dive in, it's smart to take a moment to check in with yourself. Why? Because it gives you a clear, honest picture of how you're doing right now and sets a 'baseline' to track the positive impact your new habits have over time.

On the next page is a simple chart to assess your physical and mental wellbeing. Think of it as your Midlife MOT. You can download a printable version at burningupfrozenout.com.

Sit down with your partner – each with your own chart – and score yourselves from 0 to 10 on each line. Take sleep, for example: a 0 means you didn't sleep a wink; a 10 means you leapt out of bed like the Duracell Bunny. Be honest. Talk as you go. You'll both get an instant sense of how the other's really doing.

This first week is just your starting point, so don't stress if some of the scores aren't where you'd like them to be. Over the next six weeks, aim to check in at the same time each week – ideally together, over a cup of good coffee. Update your scores, track the changes and celebrate the small wins.

Watching those numbers move in the right direction is the boost you'll need to keep going … and the proof that what you're doing is really working.

The Midlife MOT

		Week 1	Week 2	Week 3	Week 4	Week 5	Week 6
Physical health							
Overall wellbeing	How good do you feel about your overall health?						
Energy level	How energetic and alert do you feel?						
Sleep quality	How restful and refreshing is your sleep?						
Strength	How strong do you feel in your workouts or daily activities?						
Joints and muscles	How free from aches, pains or stiffness do you feel?						
Hunger levels	How balanced is your appetite (not excessive or lacking)?						
Cravings	How strong are your urges for unhealthy foods or habits?						
Digestive health	How comfortable and regular is your digestion?						
Skin health	How clear and healthy does your skin look and feel?						
Sex drive	How strong is your libido?						
Mental health							
Stress levels	How overwhelmed do you feel?						
Focus	How well can you concentrate on tasks?						
Mood	How positive are you?						
Motivation	How driven and enthusiastic do you feel?						
Cognitive sharpness	How mentally sharp and clear-headed do you feel?						
Productivity	How much have you accomplished compared to what you intended?						
Confidence	How self-assured and capable do you feel?						
Resilience	How well are you handling setbacks or challenges?						
Patience	How tolerant and understanding do you feel?						
Irritability	How easily frustrated or short-tempered are you?						
Connection with partner	How emotionally close and supported do you feel in your relationship?						
Social engagement	How connected do you feel with friends, family or colleagues?						
Sense of fun	How much joy or laughter are you experiencing?						
Sense of purpose	How meaningful and fulfilling is life?						
Gratitude levels	How much appreciation and gratitude do you have?						

It all starts with stress

With your baseline established, it's time to begin. And we're starting with stress not because it's the most important pillar, but because it's often the one that hits hardest. When you're stressed, everything else unravels faster. Sleep goes AWOL, your diet goes to hell, and exercise sounds about as appealing as assembling flat-pack furniture in a heatwave.

And if you think you're stressed – she's dealing with perimenopause, which doesn't just make stress feel worse, it also makes it biologically harder to handle.[16]

Fortunately, stress can be surprisingly quick and easy to get on top of – once you understand what's actually going on. And calming the chaos, even just a little, can trigger a ripple effect – improving your sleep, your focus, your mood, and everything else that makes life feel not just more manageable but actually enjoyable. Ready? Let's do this.

Lifestyle lifeline #1: Stress less

Put your hand up if you're stressed. Now both hands if you can't remember the last time you weren't. You're not alone, although that's cold comfort. There's no safety in numbers when it comes to sweaty-palmed panic.

Stress is the body's natural response to pressure, challenges or threats – real or imagined. And unless you're living on a desert island with no phone, no mortgage and no rolling news, you'll know modern life has turned stress from an ancient survival strategy into a full-time affliction.

That's no exaggeration: 91 percent of British adults experienced high or extreme stress in the past year, and more than one in five said they felt completely unable to manage it, according to the Mental Health UK Burnout Report 2025.[17] One in four have even had to take time off work because of poor mental health caused by pressure or stress.[18] US research paints a similarly bleak picture.[19]

We're juggling more than ever, worrying about everything from soaring bills to nuclear Armageddon. No wonder so many of us feel one small setback away from snapping. And then perimenopause shows up – uninvited and unwanted – and cranks everything up to eleven. Suddenly, stress doesn't just feel harder – it is harder.

Stress hits harder right now

During perimenopause, things she used to take in her stride can suddenly knock her for six. Why? Blame her hormones – again. Oestrogen helps regulate mood and stress response.[20] So as levels fall, so does her ability to cope, making her more sensitive to stress, anxiety and other mental health challenges.[21]

But it's not just hormonal. Perimenopause often hits during a time of shifting sands. Her body is changing in ways she can't ignore. The kids might be growing up. Ageing parents may need more care. Her career could be stalling or restarting. It's a perfect storm of pressure and uncertainty, triggering a kind of emotional and existential crisis as she enters the next chapter of her life.

It's a lot to handle. And when stress hits harder, it doesn't just drain her energy. It wrecks sleep. It kills motivation to eat well or exercise. And it pours petrol on an already raging hormonal fire – women with anxiety are up to five times more likely to suffer hot flushes and night sweats.[22]

And then boom … here comes the rage. If she's gone ballistic over something tiny – like how you loaded the dishwasher or the volume of your breathing – it's not personal. And it's more confusing and upsetting for her than it is for you.

You can't solve stress, so don't try

Think a bath bomb and scented candles will fix it? You don't get out of hot water by putting her in it.

And here's the really important bit: your job isn't to try to 'fix' her by eliminating her stress. Why? Because you can't. You'd have more luck herding cats through a car wash.

Stress is an inevitable part of life. But once you stop trying to eradicate it, you're free to focus on something far more useful – building resilience, for both of you.

And the payoff? Massive. When stress is under control, everything improves: sleep, communication, energy, even libido. She'll also have more capacity to stick with the small daily habits that ease the hormonal shitstorm now battering her brain and body.

Tune in to her stress signals

So what is your role? Tuning in to the stress you're both under. Then you can start to share the load and cut down on unnecessary daily friction – like what's for dinner, who's walking the dog, or where the hell the phone charger's gone – while building up resilience for the bigger, unavoidable stuff: rocketing inflation, relentless work deadlines, or the slow march towards our new AI overlords.

And yes, supporting someone through all this can be exhausting. If you feel helpless, rejected or like nothing you say is landing – that's OK. It's normal. You're not getting it wrong. You're simply the partner of someone going through one of the toughest life transitions there is. So, although you can't fix her stress, you can stop making it worse, and that might be the most important thing you do.

Acute vs chronic stress

Stress gets talked about like it's one thing. But it's not. There are different types,[23] but the two most people deal with day to day are acute and chronic stress. Knowing the difference matters, because it changes how you deal with it.

Acute stress	Chronic stress
Response to sudden threat	Response to constant pressures
Short-term benefits	Makes every day difficult
Body returns to normal	Long-term health problems

Acute stress is the body's short-term response to an immediate threat or challenge. Think of it like a fire alarm: loud, urgent and designed to keep you alive. It kicks in when you slam on the brakes to avoid a cyclist, sprint to catch the last train, or open your credit card bill. In small doses it can sharpen focus, boost energy and improve memory.[24] Once the moment passes, the body resets. No harm done.

Chronic stress, on the other hand, is like a faulty smoke alarm with no off switch. It's always there, buzzing away in the background, day and night. It builds up over time from ongoing demands, like money worries, work overload, relationship strain, family fallouts or health issues. It might not feel intense, but it's relentless. And that's where the damage begins.

When stress becomes chronic, the body stays stuck in a constant 'fight or flight' mode it wasn't designed for. Over time, that impacts the systems designed to keep you functioning, like sleep, mood, digestion, memory, focus, sex drive and immunity.[25] And crucially, it makes hormonal symptoms worse.[26]

Recognizing the difference between acute and chronic stress isn't just useful – it helps you spot what's really going on beneath the surface, in yourself and in your partner. And that makes it much easier to respond with empathy and practical solutions, and not frustration, avoidance or yet another argument over whose turn it is to empty the dishwasher.

Common signs of chronic stress

Chronic stress doesn't always shout – often it simmers. That makes it easy to miss, but no less harmful. And it can be even harder to spot during perimenopause, when many of the symptoms overlap or blur. Whether the root cause is hormonal or emotional, here are some of the most common signs she's on the brink:[27]

- Mood swings, snappiness or tearfulness
- Trouble falling asleep or waking through the night
- Brain fog, forgetfulness or poor concentration
- Overreacting to small frustrations
- Constant fatigue or lack of motivation
- Eating more, eating less, or craving junk food
- Pulling away from friends or family
- Saying things like 'I don't feel like myself'.

You might also notice subtle physical cues – a clenched jaw, shallow breathing, tight shoulders – that suggest her system is struggling.[28]

Meet the hormones of havoc

When the brain detects a threat, it triggers an alarm that floods the body with stress hormones that prepare you to fight, flee or freeze.[29] It's a brilliant system for dealing with immediate danger, but it's damaging when those hormones stay switched on.

Think of them like an energy drink: used at the right time, they help you focus or perform under pressure. But chugging on them all day long will leave you jumpy, wired and wide awake at night. And during perimenopause, when hormonal balance is already fragile, these stress hormones can make her symptoms worse. Here are the three main stress hormones.

Cortisol

The good: Often called the master stress hormone, cortisol helps the body deal with pressure by flooding the bloodstream with glucose for fast energy.[30] It also sharpens focus and shuts down non-essential functions like digestion, immunity and reproduction.

The bad: When cortisol levels stay high it can cause fatigue,[31] belly fat[32] and a weaker immune system,[33] as well as increase anxiety,[34] brain fog[35] and insomnia.[36]

Adrenaline

The good: Also known as epinephrine, this hormone makes your heart race, dilates your airways and redirects blood to your muscles so you're ready for action.[37]

The bad: When life feels like one emergency after another, adrenaline keeps the body in a state of high alert,[38] leading to restlessness, palpitations, jitteriness and overreactions.

Norepinephrine

The good: AKA noradrenaline, it works alongside adrenaline to heighten alertness, sharpen focus, improve reaction times and boost blood flow to the brain and muscles.[39]

The bad: Too much makes it harder to concentrate, easier to snap and almost impossible to sleep.[40]

Instant expert

Oliver Patrick on stress solutions that really work

Oliver Patrick is a physiologist and one of the UK's leading experts in lifestyle performance (oliverpatrick.com). His mission? To change the way we think about stress – not as something to avoid, but as something to master. Here are his three smart strategies for building real-world resilience, so you can handle pressure like a pro.

Stress isn't the plane, it's the pilot

Forget trying to remove stress from your life. Stress isn't the enemy – your perception of it is. The same event can feel exhilarating or overwhelming depending on your mindset. I used to hate flying. While 150 other passengers were buzzing for their holiday, I was mentally planning my funeral. If you tend to catastrophize – jumping from 'tight deadline' to 'total disaster' in seconds – you can train yourself to stop the spiral. Use visualization or mindfulness to stay present. Ask yourself: am I reacting to reality or to a disaster movie my brain's decided to direct?

Don't let a blip become a burnout

A single bad day won't break you but 35 in a row might. Your body is built to handle stress, but only when it has time to recover. Don't self-medicate with alcohol, caffeine or sugar. They might feel helpful, but they compound the problem by keeping your nervous system on high alert. After a tough day, go gentle: swap intense exercise for walking, cut back on booze and prioritize calm. That's how you stop short-term stress turning into a long-term crisis.

You need a plan, not a product

Modern wellbeing is a product marketplace. Feel anxious? Try CBD. Can't sleep? Sniff this pillow spray. No focus? Pop a nootropic. Desperation plus wishful thinking is a powerful motivator to try to spend your way out of stress, but single-issue 'solutions' won't solve the root cause. If your foundation is shaky, supplements won't fix it. Instead, build a solid base: sleep better, move more, eat well, and create calming routines with breathwork, meditation and visualization. You don't need a shopping list – you need a strategy.

Stress solutions that actually work

You instantly regretted your 'Calm down, dear!' approach to stress management, didn't you?

Remember, you can't fight stress with good intentions: suggesting she 'just relax' is as helpful as offering a cup of tea and a cuddle in the middle of a hot flush.

Here's the truth: stress isn't something you fix once – it's something you manage daily.

There are many simple, science-backed strategies that really work. Some are instant. Others take time. Some will suit you better than others. Pick what fits and ditch what doesn't. Then share them with her ... when the timing's right. A little effort goes a long way: when you're calm, you're more resilient, more switched-on, and far better equipped to create the steady, supportive space you both need.

Aromatherapy

What: Using essential oils to create a calmer mood.
Why: Scents like lavender and chamomile stimulate the brain's emotional control centre to help regulate emotions and behaviour.[41]
How: Use a diffuser or add a few drops of oil to a warm bath. Sceptical? Don't turn your nose up – it might just work.

Cognitive behavioural therapy (CBT)

What: Rewiring negative thought patterns so they don't run the show.
Why: Thoughts shape feelings and responses. If you can change the script, you can change the outcome.[42]
How: It's best done with a professional, but apps and books can help, too. Start with a simple thought diary: What happened? What did you think? Was it actually true? How could you respond next time? If she's struggling with sleep because of stress, there's a special type of CBT called CBT-I (the 'I' stands for insomnia) that can work wonders (see below).[43]

Exercise

What: Moving your body to clear your head.
Why: Physical activity releases feel-good chemicals called endorphins for greater resilience, focus and *joie de vivre*.[44]
How: Anything counts – walking, cycling, gym, dancing in the kitchen – you just have to enjoy it.

Breathwork 101

Instant calm you can carry around

Let's keep this simple: if stress is a fire alarm, breathwork is the reset button.[45] It's one of the fastest, cheapest and most effective ways to get your body out of fight-or-flight mode – the one where you're snappy, sweaty and spiralling at 3 AM – and into something far more useful: cool, calm and back in control.

And no, it's not 'just breathing'. It's intentional breathing, and it can ease anxiety, improve focus, and help you get to sleep. It's a stress-busting hack you can use anytime, anywhere – once you know how.

What is breathwork?

It's consciously changing how you breathe – typically by slowing it down, making each breath deeper, or breathing in then out in a specific pattern. The point? To use your breath to improve your mental and physical state – quickly.[46] There are many ways to do it, and you don't need anything other than a comfy chair or somewhere to lie down.

Why does it work?

Stress speeds everything up: heart rate, breathing, thoughts. Breathwork does the opposite.[47] Slowing your breath signals to your nervous system that you're safe. That triggers a cascade of calming effects: your heartbeat slows, cortisol drops, and you regain control of your emotions. The science is clear: breathwork improves mood, reduces emotional volatility, and helps you bounce back faster from sudden setbacks. Over time, it builds stress resilience – so when life throws chaos your way (or someone bursts into tears over yet another lost set of keys), you can steady the ship before it capsizes.

How to do it

Sit or lie somewhere comfortable. Relax your shoulders. Inhale through your nose (feel your lungs expand), then exhale through your mouth (feel them empty). New to breathwork? Try one of these simple techniques. A couple of minutes can make a difference. Do it first thing, sitting in traffic, once you get into bed – or anytime you feel stress start to build.

Box breathing
1 Inhale through your nose for 4 seconds.
2 Hold for 4 seconds.
3 Exhale through your mouth for 4 seconds.
4 Repeat for 2–3 minutes.
   Visualize tracing the sides of a box with each breath phase, if it helps.

4-7-8 breathing
1 Inhale through your nose for 4 seconds.
2 Hold for 7 seconds.
3 Exhale slowly through your mouth for 8 seconds.
4 Repeat for 2–4 rounds.
   Feel a bit spaced out? Perfect: that's your nervous system finally getting the memo.

Journalling

What: Writing your thoughts down so they don't rattle around your head all day.

Why: Getting it on paper clears mental clutter, short-circuits stress spirals, and helps spot unhelpful patterns and behaviours.[48]

How: Set a timer for five minutes. Write whatever comes up – frustrations, wins, weird dreams, whatever. No filter, no pressure – no one else will ever read it. Not sure where to start? Try a gratitude journal. Each night before bed, jot down one thing you're genuinely grateful for.

Meditation

What: A mental pit stop to help you pause, reflect and reset.

Why: Regular meditation lowers stress, improves focus and trains your brain to bat away anxious thoughts.[49]

How: Sit quietly and focus on your breath. When your mind wanders (and it will), simply refocus your attention. Guided meditation apps and videos are a great place to start.

Mindfulness

What: Paying full attention to what's happening now, not what might, could or should happen.

Why: It replaces judgement and self-criticism with awareness and perspective to reduce stress, anxiety and negativity.[50]

How: It's the opposite of autopilot. Notice what's around you. Listen properly. Be fully present. Meals are a great place to practise: slow down and savour the colours, smells, flavours, textures and temperature.

Progressive muscle relaxation (PMR)

What: Tensing and releasing each muscle in turn to relax your body and calm your brain.

Why: Physical tension and mental stress feed each other. PMR breaks the cycle – reducing anxiety, relieving fatigue and headaches, and improving sleep.[51]

How: Start at your feet and work your way up. Tense each muscle group for five seconds, then release for 15. Focus on the difference between tension and relaxation. It's great to do it in bed after a long day.

Sleep and social support

What: Your core foundations, alongside regular exercise and eating well.

Why: You can't out-breathe, out-meditate or out-journal bad sleep, junk food and social isolation.

How: Prioritize quality sleep (see below).[52] Find an easy and delicious way to eat (see Chapter 10). And spend more time with people who lift you up and as little time as possible with people who drag you down.[53]

> **If she's struggling, don't stay silent**
>
> If nothing is helping – and she's still overwhelmed, anxious or shutting down – it might be time to get some professional support. You don't have to handle this on your own – and neither does she. In the UK, visit mind.org or mentalhealth.org.uk. In the US, go to nami.org or adaa.org.

Relaxation 101

The stress-less day plan

You can't have a spa day five times a week, so the next best thing for keeping stress in check is structure. Just a few of these simple daily habits – and no, you don't need to do them all – can lower stress levels and make life feel calmer.

Heads-up: trying to force a stress-reduction routine on someone already frazzled will backfire faster than suggesting they 'turn that frown upside down'. The better move? Model the habits yourself. Calm is contagious: and this is your chance to lead by example.

7:00 AM Wake up wisely
Silence: Let your brain ease into the day. Ignore your phone to avoid emails, news and social media.
Sunlight: Open the curtains to calibrate your body clock and regulate stress hormones.
Hydration: Drink water before coffee to rehydrate and reduce cortisol spikes.

7:30 AM Get morning movement
Activity: Move your body for 15 minutes with walking, stretching or light exercise.
Relax: It should feel easy and enjoyable – not full-on beast mode.
Together: Invite your partner. Sunlight + movement + chat = triple win.

8:00 AM Be mindful before the mayhem
Breath: Slow, focused breathing for two minutes is a stress-busting superpower.
Focus: Set a clear intention: what's one thing you can control today?
Visualize: Picture having a calm and successful day to reduce anticipatory stress and positively prime your mind.

12:30 PM Have a midday reset
Air: A short walk or outdoor lunch break can lower stress and improve concentration.
Fuel: Prioritize protein, fibre and healthy fats over quick-fix carbs (see Chapter 10).

Inhale: Spend another couple of minutes on deep breathing before resuming work.

3:00 PM Skip the afternoon slump
Momentum: Tackle one quick, easy task to reengage focus and cut through the brain fog.
Reframe: Write down one thing – however small – that's gone well today to shift your perspective.
Posture: Stand up, stretch, then sit tall, roll your shoulders and lift your chest. Reset your body to reset your brain.

6:00 PM Transition from work to rest
Boundary: When work ends, it ends. Shut your laptop and turn off notifications.
Preparation: Work overwhelming? Write tomorrow's to-do list to clear your head.
Recovery: Take a few minutes at your desk to decompress. Breathe, stretch, listen to music.

8:30 PM Have digital downtime
Unplug: Power down screens at least one hour before bed – yes, even your phone.
Relaxation: Choose an old-school analogue activity to wind down, like reading, journalling or stretching.
Presence: Use screen-free time to reconnect with yourself or your partner.

10:00 PM Set up your sleep
Routine: A regular bedtime schedule takes the stress out of sleep (see below).
Reflection: Keep a gratitude journal and write down one thing for which you're truly grateful.
Disconnect: Dump your worries (errands, nagging thoughts, unfinished conversations) on paper and give your brain permission to switch off.

Troubleshooting stubborn stress

Some people get on the front foot at the first sign of stress. But many others take a less successful approach: they deny or downplay it … until it leaks out as cutting remarks, sarcastic comebacks, or torrential tears in the middle of IKEA.

If that sounds familiar – or you're watching your partner slowly unravel – you're not alone. But pretending everything's fine isn't a strategy. Neither is waiting for it to magically get better. And believing everyone else's needs come first – the default setting for many women – is a fast track to full-blown burnout.

So whether it's you, her or both of you caught in a stress spiral, here's how to leapfrog the most common obstacles.

Problem: I'm not stressed

Fix it: You might not feel it, but your body can't hide it. If you're wired-but-tired, struggling to sleep, or snapping over small stuff, stress is likely the quiet culprit. Same goes for her, even if she insists she's 'fine'. Signs she's not: deathly silence, sighing like she's giving CPR, or bursting into tears every time you sip your drink. Awareness is the first step towards a solution. Start simple: walk, talk, and find out how you're really doing.

Problem: Other people come first

Fix it: 'But I don't have time to be stressed!' is the unofficial mantra of midlife women everywhere. Whether she's holding down a job, holding together a household, or holding in a scream, she's too busy caring for everyone else to care for herself. Same goes for you if you're quietly trying to do it all so she doesn't have to. But you can't pour from an empty cup. Prioritizing recovery time doesn't make you selfish: it makes you happier, more present and far more useful to the people you care about.

Problem: Stress doesn't affect me

Fix it: Just because you're not shouting at the Sat Nav doesn't mean stress isn't wearing you down. Chronic stress is like a slow puncture: you might not notice it right away, but it'll leave you feeling flat as it deflates your energy, patience, sleep, and focus. Convinced you're fine? Maybe you are. But take some time out anyway – you might just notice the warning light has been flashing for a while.

Problem: I can't admit I'm struggling

Fix it: Most people would rather live without Wi-Fi than admit they're struggling with stress. But logging off from your feelings helps no one.

Being honest about your own worries or fears – however trivial they might seem – gives her permission to open up, too. And when you're talking, you can start helping each other instead of silently falling apart – individually and as a couple. Stress thrives in silence. It backs off when you say it out loud.

Problem: I don't buy into stress-busting science

Fix it: Managing stress isn't about jumping on the latest bandwagon (like ice baths), spending a small fortune (like ice baths), or pushing so far out of your comfort zone that the 'solution' is now your biggest source of stress (like ice baths). The goal is simple: find your nervous system's off switch. Try a few things that actually fit your life. Love writing? Keep a journal. Crave quiet? Try breathwork or meditation. You might only need one strategy that keeps stress in check.

Problem: I'm too overwhelmed to deal with it

Fix it: So frazzled you've just googled 'Can stress make your eye twitch'? Stress relief can often feel like one more thing on your to-do list. But the more overwhelmed you are, the more vital it is to carve out reset moments throughout the day. That's all it takes. You don't need a month-long silent retreat in Bali – just like you wouldn't fix your fitness by signing up for an ultra-marathon. Resets work best little and often.[54] Take a walk. Listen to your favourite song. Watch *The Office* bloopers on YouTube. Anything that gets you out of your head for a bit and gives your nervous system a quick time-out.

Sleep: The antidote to stress

Stress is exhausting – physically, mentally and emotionally. And the cruel irony? Just when you need rest the most, sleep is often the first casualty.[55]

But this isn't just about feeling tired. Poor sleep messes with your mood, your patience, your relationships, your body – and your ability to handle the demands of daily life.

No one should accept sleepless nights and groggy mornings as the new normal. Sleep isn't a luxury – it's a launchpad. When you both get the rest you need, everything feels easier. The clouds part. Energy soars. Mood lifts. Libido returns.

And no, this isn't about perfect sleep every night. Just a few smart tweaks to what you're already doing can change everything.

Lifestyle lifeline #2: Sleep better

Tired? Of course you are. Welcome to midlife, where sleep gets harder the more you need it.

Back in the day, you'd be all over each other at 1 AM – hot, sweaty and swearing there'd be no sleep for hours (well, five more minutes, at least). These days, the nights are still hot and sweaty, but the swearing's under your breath as you both stare at the ceiling in silence and mentally scroll through tomorrow's to-do list.

Sleep: The pillar that supports everything

Not getting enough sleep doesn't just make you tired – it disrupts your mood, memory, metabolism, motivation, and just about every other biological system.[56]

We said at the start of this chapter that sleep was one of the big four lifestyle pillars – alongside stress management, eating, and exercise – that support a healthy, happy and long life.

But here's the truth: sleep isn't just a pillar. It's the foundation the others are built on.

If you're sleeping badly, it's harder to eat well, move your body, think clearly or even be nice to the people you love. Everything – even brushing your teeth – feels as exhausting as doing the bleep test on a sandy beach.

Mayhem, mood swings and midnight meltdowns

For many women in perimenopause, sleep is a big problem.[57] Falling oestrogen levels interfere with how her body regulates its temperature, stress response, mood and more – all of which affect her ability to fall and then stay asleep.

In fact, up to 60 percent of perimenopausal and postmenopausal women report suffering from insomnia, which includes difficulty falling asleep, staying asleep and waking up too early.[58]

Even if her sleep routine once ran like clockwork, now it's more like a rail replacement bus service: frustrating, uncomfortable, and no guarantee when it'll arrive – if at all.

And for men? We have our own midlife sleep saboteurs: stress, work, money ... and now that small-hour need to pee.

Even if you've always slept just fine, a hibernating bear isn't the emotional support animal she needs right now. So, if she's not sleeping, don't expect to either. Her sleep problem is now your sleep problem. So, if you've started wondering whether a bunkbed might be the answer, good news: there's no need to fall out over whose turn it is to go on top.

Sleep FAQ: What it is and why you need it

Before we dive into the fixes, here are the answers to the most common questions – so you can spot what you're nailing and where things might be coming unstuck.

What is sleep?

Sleep is your brain and body's auto-repair system.[59] While you're in the Land of Nod, it's hard at work: processing memories, repairing muscle tissue, regulating your immune, hormonal and metabolic systems, and powering through a million other essential tasks you've probably never even thought about.

Why do we sleep?

We still don't fully understand why we sleep, only that without it everything goes wrong – fast. Your immune system struggles.[60] Your mood nosedives. You gain weight.[61] You lose energy, motivation and libido. Sleep supports every aspect of your physical, mental and emotional health.[62]

How much sleep do I need?

Most adults need between seven and nine hours a night.[63] If you're under a lot of stress or physically pushing yourself, you may need more.[64,65] Some people get by on less, but most of us start showing signs of sleep deprivation after a few bad nights.[66] And no, mainlining caffeine isn't a viable solution (see below).[67]

How do I know if I'm getting enough?

You probably aren't, but here's how to tell for sure. If you wake up groggy, rely on caffeine to get going, struggle to focus, snap more than usual, or regularly forget why you walked into a room, you're likely sleep-deprived. Smartwatches and sleep trackers can help you spot patterns, but don't get too hung up on the data – obsessing over sleep scores can actually make things worse.[68] The real test? Are you jumping out of bed ready to seize the day or hitting snooze for the umpteenth time?

What happens if I don't fix it?

You can get away with the odd bad night. But string together enough of them and the problems stack up. The short-term symptoms – more colds, worse moods, constant anxiety – are bad enough. The long-term health risks are far more serious: ongoing sleep deprivation raises your risk of depression, heart disease, diabetes and dementia.[69] That said, poor sleep itself won't kill you, and worrying about it often makes things worse. In fact, fear of not sleeping is a very common cause of insomnia. But there are proven ways to break that cycle – and it's easier than you might think (see below).

How can I get better sleep?

You have to get the basics right. Get sunlight in the morning.[70] Cut screen time in the evening.[71] Keep your bedroom cool, quiet and dark.[72] Stick to regular sleep and wake times – even on weekends.[73] And avoid anything that spikes stress before bed, like checking emails, watching the news, or resuming last year's tax return.[74] Oh – and you already know this – sex can help (see Chapter 12).[75] Oxytocin (the cuddle hormone) and prolactin (the satisfaction hormone) both promote sleep.[76] So if you're struggling to drift off, you've got options ...

What if nothing seems to be working?

Tried everything yet still wide awake at stupid o'clock? Cognitive behavioural therapy for insomnia (CBT-I) is one of the best treatments for sleep problems.[77] It works by tackling the unhelpful thoughts and behaviours behind poor sleep, especially when stress or hormones are involved.[78] You can do it with a therapist or through guided online sessions, and the benefits can be permanent.[79]

Can you sleep too much?

It sounds idyllic, but regularly clocking nine-plus hours and still waking up knackered means something's up.[80] It could be a sign of an underlying issue like depression, chronic fatigue or another health condition. Speak to your GP: your body might not need more sleep, just more support.

6 ways to get sensational sleep

Still closing your eyes and hoping for the best? You've got more control than you think. Here's how to stop chasing sleep and start catching it:

1 **Have a sleep schedule.** Wake up and go to bed at the same time every day. Even weekends. Doing so helps you fall asleep faster and spend more time in the more restorative stages of sleep.
2 **Start the day with sunshine.** Sunlight is the number-one regulator of your body clock that instructs the wake–sleep cycle. Get outside for 20 minutes in the morning and again in the afternoon as often as you can.
3 **Switch off your screens.** Artificial light in the evening blocks the release of melatonin, the hormone that promotes sleepiness. Blue light – the type emitted from phones, tablets and TVs – is especially bad. Switch off all screens at least an hour before bed.
4 **De-stress for deeper sleep.** The best stress-busting strategies are the ones that fit into your day without adding more pressure. Journaling is especially effective, as is breathwork. Small, repeatable habits always beat occasional grand gestures.
5 **Time your dinner right.** Big, late-night meals rev up your digestive system, which can delay sleep. Eat dinner at least one hour before bed, and avoid especially fatty or spicy foods.
6 **Set the scene for sleep.** Keep the bedroom cool (20–25°C, or 68–77°F, is ideal – though she may prefer it cooler), dark (use blackout blinds or an eye mask), and quiet (try earplugs or white noise). Clear any clutter – your brain unwinds faster in a tidy room – and avoid using your bedroom for work or TV. Beds are for sex and sleep, not Netflix and notifications.

Coffee and cocktails: The sleep saboteurs

A double espresso to get going, a glass of wine to wind down – sound familiar? The trouble is, both caffeine and alcohol could be the reason you're wired at bedtime and staring at the ceiling all night. Here's what's going on and what to drink instead.

Caffeine is great for a morning boost but a disaster for your bedtime routine.[81] It blocks the build-up of sleep pressure (that natural drive to fall asleep the longer you're awake), lingers in your system for hours, and disrupts deep sleep even if you do nod off.[82] Cut all caffeine after lunchtime – not just coffee and tea, but cola and energy drinks too – if you want to sleep better tonight.

Alcohol might help you crash out quickly, but it's a sleep thief in disguise. It disrupts REM sleep[83] (the restorative dream phase) and makes those witching hour wake-ups[84] – often filled with spiralling fears, existential dread and a highlight reel of every mistake you've ever made – far more likely. Alcohol-free beers and spirits are now pretty decent (wine's still hit-and-miss) if you want to go booze-free or alternate with zero percent options.

Swap night sweats for sweet dreams

Hot flushes and night sweats are among the most common menopause symptoms and the most likely to wreck her sleep. Whether she can't drift off because she's roasting or wakes up drenched every night, here's what can help.

1 **Divvy up the duvets.** Still want to share a bed? Try the Scandinavian sleep method: swap one big duvet for two smaller ones – with different togs if needed – so she can control her temperature without freezing your nuts off.[85]
2 **Favour natural fabrics.** Synthetic bedding and pyjamas trap heat and moisture like a greenhouse. Switch to breathable natural fibres – cotton, linen or bamboo – for sheets, duvet covers and nightwear that wick moisture and prevent overheating.[86]
3 **Blow off some steam.** A bedside fan or open window can help – just open it early in the evening to let the heat escape. Still too hot? Cooling pillows,[87] gel mats[88] and smart mattress covers[89] can regulate body temperature, ease night sweats and improve sleep quality.

4. **Supplement her sleep.** Magnesium glycinate may help ease hot flushes by promoting relaxation and lowering core body temperature[90] – and it's less likely to cause stomach issues than other forms. Always check with a GP before starting any new supplement.
5. **Don't take it personally.** If she demands you sleep in another bed (or hemisphere), support her without sulking – even if you end up on the sofa. Her symptoms aren't a reflection on you – and if you stick with it, the tips in this chapter (and the next) should help turn down the temperature (and the tension) several degrees.

To nap or not to nap?

Flagging after lunch? A short afternoon nap can boost energy, focus and mood,[91] lower stress,[92] and even improve heart health,[93] but nap too long[94] or too late[95] and it'll come back to haunt you at bedtime. So if you're working from home, go for it. In the office? Best to power through: unless you're the boss, it might cause more problems than it solves.

Cap your nap at 30 minutes to avoid sleep inertia (that foggy, just-woke-up feeling), and make sure you're up before 3 PM so it doesn't sabotage your night. A dark, quiet room helps, as do an eye mask and earplugs. And don't forget to set an alarm.

Instant expert

Nick Littlehales on how even insomniacs can sleep better
Nick Littlehales is a world-renowned sleep coach and author of Sleep: The myth of 8 hours, The power of naps ... and the new plan to recharge your body and mind.[96] *His innovative approach ditches one-size-fits-all rules in favour of smart, science-backed strategies (sportsleepcoach.com). Here are his five tips to help even lifelong night owls drift off without any drama.*

Don't obsess over eight hours
Most people can't manage eight hours of uninterrupted sleep, and that's OK. Sleep works in 90-minute cycles, so start thinking in terms of

cycles, not hours. Try aiming for five cycles (7.5 hours), but four (6 hours) can be enough if you build in recovery during the day (see below). Only managed three cycles? Don't panic! What matters most is consistency over the week – not perfection every night.

Rise early every day

Your wake-up time is your daily anchor. Pick one – ideally near sunrise – and stick to it, even after a rough night. Start the day with daylight, movement and hydration: open the curtains, drink a glass of water, stretch or go for a ten-minute walk. This simple routine acts as a full body-clock reset to get your rhythm back on track. Don't hit snooze. Get up, get going, and you'll sleep better tonight.

Awake at night? Don't fight the fear

Waking up at night isn't a failure – it's actually pretty normal. The real problem is the panic that comes with it. If you can't get back to sleep after 20 minutes, don't just lie there stewing. Get up quietly, keep the lights low, and do something calm that's not overly stimulating: reading or journaling, stretching or prepping food, not Netflix or Instagram. Give your brain space to reset, then go back for another sleep cycle. You'll sleep far better when you stop trying to force it.

Recover during the day

Your brain isn't built to go full throttle all day long. Every 90 minutes, take a five-minute break. Step away from your screen, go outside or sit quietly for breathwork or meditation. These micro recovery moments (MRMs) help reduce stress and rebalance your rhythm, which takes the pressure off bedtime. Set a timer if it helps, and treat your MRMs as sacrosanct. They're as important as anything else in your diary.

Treat sleep as a 24-hour habit

A blackout blind and an expensive mattress won't save your sleep if the rest of your day is out of sync. What matters most is the rhythm of your day: when and how you wake, eat, move, rest and recover. So yes, a cool, dark and quiet bedroom helps, but don't obsess over the perfect set-up or make your pre-bed routine another source of stress. Sleep isn't a performance – it's a pattern.

From surviving to thriving

When you're stressed and sleep-deprived, everything feels like an ordeal – work, chores, even deciding what to have for dinner.

But calm your mind and give your body the rest it needs, and everything changes. Get the sleep and stress pieces in place, and suddenly you've got more energy, more motivation, and the drive to keep that virtuous circle turning.

Now, the idea of eating better or moving more doesn't feel like climbing Everest in flip-flops. It feels possible. Maybe even exciting.

In the next chapters, we'll show you how to build smarter habits around food and fitness – without the grind, guesswork or grim green sludge smoothies – so you're not simply surviving midlife, you're smashing it.

10

Eat smarter
Good mood food for hormones, health and happiness

We've tackled stress and sleep – the two silent saboteurs of midlife health, and the biggest barriers to feeling calm, clear-headed and in control. Now the focus is on food. Because what you eat – and how you eat it – can transform how you both look, feel and function.

And it's not about rules, restrictions or rabbit food. It's about smart, satisfying choices that fit seamlessly into your life. You'll learn how to make food your friend – for your hormones, your brain and your body.

This isn't about eating less. It's about eating smarter. Enjoying meals that support your energy, muscle, metabolism and mental health. With a few simple swaps, you can both enjoy the kind of food that fuels your best life – without any faff, fads or fuss.

In this chapter you'll discover:

- The science-backed way to eat for weight loss, energy and longevity
- How protein fights fat, protects muscle and keeps her strong
- Simple ways to eat well without banning the food you love
- Why emotional eating strikes, and what to do when it does
- The real impact of alcohol on sleep, hormones and mood
- Which supplements are worth it, and why some are a waste of money
- Why gut health matters more than ever, and how to improve hers (and yours).

Lifestyle lifeline #3: Eat smarter

You are what you eat.

Actually, you're what you absorb, and we'll get to the gut, and its surprisingly big impact on your health and happiness, shortly (see below).

The food we eat – and how much of it – has a huge bearing on how we look and feel, especially in midlife. Long gone are the days when you could eat (and drink) whatever you wanted without gaining an ounce of fat.[1]

But here's the thing: eating for a healthier body and a happier mind is much easier than you think. You don't have to ban hundreds of foods. You don't need to drink concoctions that look – and smell – like they've come out the back of your lawnmower. And you don't have to cross the road every time you see the Golden Arches.

Healthy eating made easy

What you do need is an eating approach that follows two golden rules: it must suit your tastes and food preferences; and it must be easy and enjoyable enough to stick with for the foreseeable, without making you dread mealtimes.

And that's where most people go wrong. They jump on restrictive, joyless diets that promise miracles but are impossible to sustain, so they crash, then binge.[2] The result? Weight gain instead of weight loss,[3] with a side serving of guilt, misery and shame.[4]

Before we get into the smart, sustainable eating strategies that will make you healthier and happier, let's first look at what your meals are actually made of.

Meet the macros

All food is made up of one or more of the three main macronutrients: carbohydrates, protein and fat. These 'macros' are the nutrients your body needs in large amounts every day to fuel essential functions, keep you healthy, and help you feel and perform at your best.[5]

Carbohydrates

- boost energy
- lift mood
- reduce stress.

Protein

- builds muscle
- controls cravings
- speeds recovery.

Fats

- support brain health
- make hormones
- absorb vitamins.

Carbohydrates are your body's go-to source of fuel, providing four calories per gram.[6] They come in two forms: simple carbs (sugars), which are absorbed quickly for an instant energy hit, and complex carbs (wholegrains, beans and starchy veg), which contain fibre and release energy more slowly and steadily. For most people, carbs should make up around 45–65 percent of total daily calories – ideally from complex sources.[7]

Protein isn't just for building muscle – it provides four calories per gram and is essential for tissue repair, immune function, and the production of enzymes and hormones.[8] During perimenopause, it becomes even more important to preserve muscle mass and bone strength.[9] Animal-based sources like red meat, poultry, fish and eggs are complete proteins because they contain all nine essential amino acids. Plant-based sources – lentils, chickpeas, nuts, seeds and grains – are incomplete, but can be combined to meet your needs. Depending on activity levels, protein should account for 10–35 percent of daily calories.[10]

Fat gets a bad rap – mostly because it's the most energy-dense macronutrient, delivering nine calories per gram – but it's crucial for hormone production, brain health and nutrient absorption.[11] It comes in three main types: unsaturated fats (found in avocados, olive oil, nuts and oily fish) are the healthiest and should make up the bulk of your intake. Saturated fats (from meat and full-fat dairy) are fine in moderation. Trans fats – found in ultra-processed snacks and some fast food – are best avoided. Ideally, fats should make up 20–35 percent of your daily calories.[12]

Protein 101

Power up to slow down ageing

You don't lose muscle because you get old: you get old because you lose muscle.

That's why so many women – and men – feel weaker, wobblier and more worn out in midlife. As hormones dip, so does muscle mass. Strength slips, energy slumps and belly fat moves in. But it's not inevitable.

The fix? More protein. Why? It's your body's building blocks – it keeps muscles strong, bones dense, energy steady, appetite in check and your immune system firing.

In the UK, the daily recommendation intake is 0.75g of protein per kilogram of bodyweight, which works out at just 45g a day for a 60kg (132lb) woman.[13] In the US, the advice is 0.8g per kilo.[14]

The problem? During perimenopause that won't touch the sides.

Some women rarely fancy protein-packed foods. Others feel too full afterwards. And there's still that myth that protein makes her bulky – it doesn't.[15]

Protein is her pension

Your job? Help her realize the truth: every bite is a deposit into her future strength, energy and independence – especially if she's lifting weights (see Chapter 4).

So how much protein does she actually need? Around 1–1.2g per kilo of bodyweight.[16] Aim for three meals with 20–25g of protein each to get the job done.

The best sources include lean red meat, fish, chicken, turkey, eggs, Greek yoghurt, tofu, lentils, beans, quinoa and nuts. If she's mostly plant-based, pair grains and legumes to get all the essential amino acids.[17]

So she can forget the fancy anti-ageing creams, potions and lotions – protein's the best way to turn back the clock.

Turning macros into meals

Knowing about macros is one thing, but how do you turn them into a way of eating that supports better health and happiness? Like many things in life, there's no one-size-fits-all solution – only the approach that works best for you. That means choosing a way of eating that's simple, satisfying and sustainable – and one you can stick with long term, because it's delicious and aligned with your personal preferences, values and lifestyle.

The diets that deliver

Want a smarter way to eat – one that boosts energy, supports hormonal and overall health, and still lets you enjoy your food? These tried-and-tested approaches are a great place to start. They focus on unprocessed, nutrient-dense foods and are simple enough to stick with for the long haul.

Mediterranean diet: Rich in fresh fruits and vegetables, unprocessed wholegrains, healthy fats and lean animal protein, with an emphasis on social eating.[18]

DASH diet: Designed to lower blood pressure, it prioritizes whole foods, lean protein and a reduced salt intake.[19]

Flexitarian diet: Primarily plant-based but allows for occasional meat and fish, making it flexible and balanced.[20]

Nordic diet: Similar to the Mediterranean diet but adapted to Northern European foods and features more fatty fish and root vegetables.[21]

Pescatarian diet: Primarily plant-based but includes fish, seafood, dairy and eggs.[22]

Vegetarian diet: Primarily plant-based and excludes all animal meat but may include dairy and eggs for protein.[23]

Vegan diet: Exclusively plant-based and excludes all animal-derived products and requires careful planning to avoid any nutritional deficiencies, including protein.[24]

Don't fall for these food fads

These so-called 'quick fix' diets are popular because they promise rapid weight loss – but they're hard to sustain, often lacking in essential nutrients, and almost always lead to weight regain once you stop. The result? More stress, greater frustration – and you end up back at square one.

Keto diet: Extremely low-carb, high-fat diet that requires meticulous planning and may lead to nutrient deficiencies, digestive issues and heart disease.[25]

Carnivore diet: A more restrictive type of keto diet: only animal meat is allowed so it's high in saturated fat and low in fibre and other essential nutrients.[26]

Cambridge diet: A very low-calorie meal replacement diet that often leads to weight regain when it ends.[27]

Juice cleanses and detox diets: Low in protein and calories, they often lead to energy crashes, rapid weight regain and eating disorders.[28]

Very low-calorie diets (VLCDs): Extreme calorie restriction that can slow metabolism and lead to muscle loss.[29]

Food-named diets (e.g. cabbage soup diet): Overly restrictive, nutritionally unbalanced,[30] and guaranteed to give you the kind of farts that clear a room faster than a fire alarm.

Head to the Med

If there's one way of eating that most nutrition experts recommend and scientific research supports during midlife – especially around perimenopause – it's the Mediterranean diet.[31] Why? It's simple, sustainable and backed by a library of studies for its health benefits.[32]

It's not actually a diet in the traditional sense – more flexible eating guidelines centred on fresh vegetables, healthy fats, unprocessed carbs, lean protein and shared, social meals. Oh, and it happens to be delicious. Here's what you need to know.

What is the Mediterranean diet?

Inspired by the eating habits of countries around the Mediterranean Sea – including Spain, Italy and Greece – the Med diet has gained global popularity for its proven health and longevity benefits.[33]

Unlike most diets, which focus on rules and restriction, it's relaxed, flexible and focused on enjoying whole foods in a sociable setting.

What's in the Mediterranean diet?

It's rich in plant-based foods, healthy fats and lean protein and low in added sugar and processed ingredients.[34] That means plenty of fresh fruit and veg, wholegrains, legumes, nuts, seeds, and protein from fish and seafood. You'll also find moderate amounts of yoghurt and cheese, the occasional serving of red meat, and herbs and spices used instead of salt to add flavour. Olive oil is the star of the show: its high monounsaturated fat content[35] can help reduce inflammation[36] and lower heart disease risk,[37] while its polyphenol antioxidants[38] offer protection against cancer[39] and cognitive decline.[40]

Instant expert

Nigel Denby on eating for greater health and happiness

Nigel Denby is a registered dietitian, author[41] and broadcaster, and one of the UK's leading voices on midlife nutrition (harleystathome.com). His philosophy? To cut through the diet nonsense and show women how to eat well, feel better and take back control – one delicious meal at a time.

Pack your plate with protein

Protein from nuts, seeds, fish and meat helps maintain and build muscle, strengthens bones, and supports healthy ageing by reducing the risk of osteoporosis. It also takes longer to digest than carbs or fat, keeping you fuller for longer. On top of that, it balances blood sugar to prevent energy crashes and boosts production of key brain chemicals like dopamine and serotonin – improving mood, focus and mental clarity.

Fill up with fibre

Fibre also helps you feel fuller for longer, which reduces snacking and supports weight management. It also stabilizes blood sugar to help prevent insulin resistance – a major cause of type-2 diabetes. Just as importantly, it feeds the gut bacteria involved in hormone metabolism and immune defence, and helps lower cholesterol to reduce your risk of heart disease. Aim for at least 30g a day – nearly double the 17g most of us currently manage.

Love heart-healthy fats

Healthy fats – especially omega-3s from oily fish and monounsaturated fats from olive oil – support brain and heart health, boosting cognitive function and lowering disease risk. Fats also play a vital role in hormone production, help reduce inflammation linked to pain and chronic illness, and aid the absorption of vitamins needed for a healthy metabolism, immune system, skin and cardiovascular function.

Eat the rainbow

Fruits and vegetables are packed with antioxidants, vitamins, minerals and plant compounds that fight inflammation, protect your heart, and boost overall wellbeing. Different foods contain different nutrients, so aim for variety: try to eat at least 30 – yes, 30 – different coloured fruits and veg each week. And don't stress about fresh – frozen is just as good.

Make every meal a moment

Food isn't just fuel – especially in the Mediterranean approach, where meals are a chance to connect with others over lovingly prepared, delicious dishes. Sharing food encourages slower, more mindful eating that you actually savour, instead of the rushed, mindless overeating that happens when you're slumped on the sofa in front of the TV.

A day on the Med diet

You've seen the benefits, but what does it look like in practice? Here's a sample day's menu to show how simple (and delicious) it can be. Get free weekly meal plans and recipes to make healthy eating a no-brainer at burningupfrozenout.com.

Breakfast: Scrambled eggs with feta and cherry tomatoes on wholegrain toast, with a handful of almonds
Lunch: Grilled lemon and herb chicken breast with a quinoa and roasted vegetable salad, drizzled with extra-virgin olive oil
Snack: Hummus with carrot and cucumber sticks, with a handful of olives
Dinner: Grilled sea bass with roasted new potatoes, sautéed spinach and garlic-roasted cherry tomatoes

Instant expert

Rhiannon Lambert on making mealtimes tasty, fun and easy

Rhiannon Lambert is one of the UK's top nutritionists, a Sunday Times best-selling author,[42] and founder of Rhitrition – a leading nutrition clinic and consultancy (rhitrition.com). She cuts through the confusion to help people eat well without overthinking it. Quick, balanced and genuinely delicious, her five fast-food rules will save you time, money and stress.

Start small

Overhauling your diet overnight is overwhelming and very hard to sustain. Instead, make small, gradual changes that add up over time. Start by adding extra vegetables to meals, swapping sugary cereals for porridge, fruit and nut butter, or choosing fibre-full wholegrains like brown rice over processed white pasta. These simple shifts create lasting habits – without the pressure of perfection.

Upgrade, don't eliminate

You don't have to give up your favourite meals, just find healthier versions. Swap takeaway fish and chips for grilled fish with homemade oven-baked chips, or make pizza using wholegrain flour with veggie toppings. By upgrading familiar favourites rather than eliminating them entirely, you can enjoy balanced eating without feeling deprived or restricted.

Be adventurous

Many people assume they dislike certain foods simply because they've never tried them or not had them in years. Our taste preferences change over time, and experimenting with different flavours and textures can make healthy eating more enjoyable. Not a fan of vegetables? Try cooking them in new ways – roasting, steaming or grilling – and adding fresh herbs and spices can transform their taste and texture. And try lentils, chickpeas or tofu for extra plant-based protein.

Plan meals together

When both partners are involved in meal planning it's easier to create meals that suit different tastes. Set aside time each week to choose recipes, make a shopping list, and order food online. This helps you stick to your budget, avoid impulse purchases, and ensure you buy only what you need – rather than making less healthy choices when you shop hungry.

Cook once, eat all week

Batch cooking is a game-changer for busy couples. Preparing extra portions of protein-rich meals means you'll always have nutritious options ready to go. Freezer-friendly lunches and dinners like soups, stews and curries make weeknight dinners quick and effortless and reduce expensive food waste. Take turns cooking, or do it as a team: it's a great way to eat better and spend quality time together.

Food fix #1: 6 ways to avoid overeating without going hungry

Of course, it's not just what you eat that matters. How, when and why you eat also affect your weight and how good you look, feel and perform.

Overeating is a leading cause of weight gain,[43] but it's rarely down to a lack of willpower – it's about habits, hormones, and having too much on your plate (both figuratively and literally).[44] With a few simple tweaks, you can both feel more in control around food – without the effort, frustration or guilt.

Problem 1: Portion creep

Eating similar portions as you (who has more muscle and needs more fuel) or teenage kids (who burn through energy faster than cans of body spray) means those extra calories add up over time.[45]

Solve it: *Downsize without sacrifice*

Using smaller bowls or plates can help reduce portion size without it feeling stingy.[46] Med-style meals encourage smaller servings of nutrient-dense foods, so dinner still feels generous and satisfying – just without the belt-busting platefuls.

Problem 2: Mindless munching

Dinner gets demolished between answering emails, breaking up sibling squabbles and bingeing *Bake Off* episodes. She barely remembers what she had, but her plate's spotless – and she's still peckish. So she goes back for round two. And three.

Solve it: *Take it to the table*

Ditch the screens and sit at the table.[47] Chat. Chew. Savour. The best meals aren't just about what's on the plate – they're about presence, pacing and pleasure. When you're tuned in, you notice when you're full and stop before you're stuffed.

Problem 3: Weekend blowouts

Restriction leads to rebellion.[48] So if you've been 'good' all week, Friday night's a free-for-all: crisps, booze, takeaway, ice cream, the works.

Solve it: *Treat the week as a whole*

Med-style meals – with lots of tasty stuff in moderate amounts – remove the need for weekend blowouts. A glass of red with dinner, a little cheese, a square of dark chocolate when the mood hits. If nothing's banned, nothing gets binged.

Problem 4: 'Saving up' calories

Think skipping breakfast and lunch is the best way to lose weight?[49] Then why, by mid-afternoon, does the fridge get cleaned out like an Amazon warehouse on Black Friday?

Solve it: *Keep the tank fuelled*

Three meals a day – each with protein, fibre and healthy fats – is the best way to steady blood sugar and prevent binges.[50] Peckish before dinner? Have a handful of nuts.[51]

Problem 5: All-or-nothing thinking

One biscuit = day ruined = might as well scoff the whole packet.[52]

Solve it: Reset and move on
One biscuit is just that – not a moral failing. Slip-ups don't derail progress – staying stuck in them does. Take a breath, refocus and move on.[53] A short walk can quickly reset your mindset.[54]

Problem 6: Underestimating liquid calories
Lattes, smoothies, wine and juices aren't filling like food, but the calories still count.[55] And they're so easy to over-consume.[56]

Solve it: Sip smarter
Ditch abstinence for awareness. A milky coffee or glass of wine has its place – ideally alongside a slow, satisfying meal. But guzzling sugar-laden drinks all day piles on the pounds.[57] Sparkling water,[58] green tea[59] or black coffee[60] are smart, satisfying swaps.

> ### Emotional eating: When food becomes the fix
> We don't eat just because we're hungry. Sometimes it's because we're stressed, sad, bored or completely overwhelmed.
>
> That's emotional eating,[61] and during perimenopause, it can hit harder than ever.[62] No surprise there – food brings fast, easy comfort, at least in the moment.
>
> But this isn't about willpower – it's about awareness. Next time she's about to inhale a packet of crisps, suggest something else – or better still, do it together. Talk. Walk. Hold the punch bag while she knocks seven bells out of it.[63] Anything that tackles the stress better than raiding the biscuit tin.[64] If it's chocolate she really wants? That's fine too – if it's a conscious choice and not a coping mechanism on autopilot. Food can be a real comfort – but not if it leaves you feeling worse afterwards.

Food fix #2: 7 ways to curb cravings without going crazy

Cravings are intense urges to eat sugary, salty or fatty foods – it's never kale, is it? – and they often have little to do with being hungry. They're driven by a mix of biology (Hi, hormones![65]), psychology (Hi, stress![66]), and habit (Hi, 10 AM biscuit tin![67]).

Eat smarter

Cravings can feel relentless[68] during perimenopause,[69] but they don't stand a chance when she's got a plan. Here's how to outsmart them the easy way.

1. **Drink water first.** Dehydration can mimic hunger – you may be thirsty, not starving.[70] Drink a big glass of water, wait 10 minutes, and the craving will probably pass.[71]
2. **Prioritize protein and fibre.** Build meals around these two – remember, they keep you fuller for longer[72] and help stabilize blood sugar,[73] stopping the dips that spark snack attacks.
3. **Don't skip meals.** Going too long without food sends blood sugar into free fall,[74] and that's when cravings hit hardest.[75] Regular meals and smart snacks help keep hunger (and hanger) at bay.[76]
4. **Swap, don't stop.** Craving crisps? Try salted popcorn – all the crunch, far less fat.[77] Love chocolate? Go dark: 70 percent cocoa or higher is full of antioxidants.[78] Fancy ice cream? Greek yoghurt with frozen fruit (sliced banana is especially good) hits the spot and packs protein.[79] Upgrades beat deprivation every time.
5. **Know your triggers.** Tired? Stressed? Bored? That's when sweets call like sirens. Give your body what it actually needs: a stretch, a chat, five quiet minutes or some fresh air – a change of scenery can crush most cravings.[80]
6. **Don't ban your favourites.** Banning your favourite foods makes you fixate on them until you cave in and overdo it.[81] A little bit of what you fancy now and then satisfies your sweet tooth. Eaten mindfully, you'll savour every second.[82]
7. **Clear out the cupboards.** If it's not in the house, it can't call your name at 9 PM. Avoid food shopping when hungry[83] and stock up on smarter snacks – think nuts, yoghurt, fruit or seeds – so there's always a better option to hand.

Alcohol 101

Just how bad is booze?

You knew this was coming, didn't you? Let's start with the reality: alcohol isn't good for you – in any amount. A 25-year study of drinking habits in 195 countries, published in *The Lancet*, found that no level of consumption was safe. Even small amounts raise the risk of heart disease and cancer.[84]

In fact, alcohol is officially classified as a Group 1 carcinogen by the International Agency for Research on Cancer (up there with asbestos and tobacco) because of its link to several cancers, including breast cancer in women and bowel cancer in men.[85] It also increases the risk of liver damage,[86] heart problems[87] and cognitive decline.[88] For women, it can make perimenopause symptoms like hot flushes and night sweats worse,[89] and can increase the risk of osteoporosis[90] and heart disease.[91]

That's the science. Here's the reality: most people don't want to be teetotal. And that's OK.

We're not here to tell you what to do – just give you the clearest, most up-to-date evidence so you can make informed decisions that feel right for you. Cutting back, even a bit, can protect her health, help her sleep better[92] and save you a small fortune in the process.

And yes, wine is part of the Mediterranean lifestyle. But there's a big difference between a glass of Rioja with a slow, sociable dinner and six pints of Stella down the Dog and Duck every night. As with most things in life, balance is everything – especially when it comes to booze.

Gut instinct: Why the menopause messes with digestion

Many women suddenly experience bloating, constipation, diarrhoea and other digestive discomfort in perimenopause, even if they've never had gut issues before.[93] The reason? Oestrogen – obviously.[94]

The digestive system is packed with oestrogen receptors.[95] When hormone levels decline, the delicate brain–gut connection is knocked out of whack, affecting digestion. Increased stress and anxiety can also impair digestive function.[96]

These symptoms generally don't meet the diagnostic threshold for IBS, but they can be just as distressing and just as disruptive.

Some women experience more severe symptoms than others, and one possible reason is how efficiently their body reabsorbs oestrogen.[97] After being processed by the liver, oestrogen is sent into bile and excreted via bowel movements. But certain gut microbes produce enzymes that can reactivate it, allowing some to be reabsorbed into the bloodstream.

Women with a gut microbiome that supports this process may retain more oestrogen,[98] easing menopausal symptoms. Others lose more, leading to a sharper hormonal drop and more severe digestive and overall health problems.

If she's really struggling, some simple diet and lifestyle tweaks can help rebalance digestion, support microbial diversity and improve oestrogen reabsorption – all of which can ease symptoms.

Instant expert

Professor Emeran Mayer's fast fixes for a happier, healthier gut

Emeran Mayer is a world-renowned gastroenterologist whose pioneering work has transformed our understanding of the gut–brain connection (emeranmayer.com). His decades of research reveal how the gut microbiome influences everything from hormone balance and mood to inflammation, immunity and even longevity.[99] Here's his science-backed advice for better digestion, lower stress, and greater health and happiness.

Focus on fibre

Fibre is crucial for healthy digestion, gut microbial health, stable blood sugar and the prevention of gut inflammation, but most of us don't eat enough. Aim for 30–40g daily, slowly increasing your intake to avoid bloating and discomfort. Adding a variety of more vegetables, legumes and whole grains over time gives your gut the chance to adapt.

Feed your gut

A thriving gut microbiome loves variety. Aim for at least 30 different plant-based foods each week – vegetables, fruits, legumes, nuts, seeds and wholegrains – to boost diversity. A more varied diet doesn't just improve digestion, it may also help her body reabsorb more oestrogen, easing menopause symptoms.

Eat fermented foods

Naturally fermented foods like sauerkraut, kimchi, kombucha and kefir have been shown to boost microbial diversity. Unlike most mass-produced probiotic drinks and yoghurts (often loaded with sugar, additives and overblown health claims), fermented foods deliver beneficial bacteria in their purest, most potent form.

Ditch processed food

Ultra-processed foods (UPFs) are packed with sugar, emulsifiers, artificial sweeteners, food dyes and preservatives that disrupt the gut microbiome. If the label reads like a chemistry set of unpronounceable ingredients, it's ultra-processed and best avoided.

Solve stress

Food is only part of the picture. Chronic stress wreaks havoc on the health of the gut and its microbiome via the brain–gut–microbiome connection, disturbing the gut microbial ecosystem, increasing gut permeability – or 'leaky gut' – and triggering inflammation. A few minutes of focused breathing is a fast, free and effective way to calm your mind and soothe your digestive system.

Are supplements the solution?

If only.

Walk into any health food shop and you'll see shelves stacked with products promising to fix almost any ailment. The problem? Supplements are a bit like politicians: full of big promises, light on real results.

Still, health pills are big business. The global supplement market was worth a whopping £138 billion ($178 billion) in 2023,[100] with around $17 billion splurged on menopause-related products alone.[101]

Driven by influencer hype, social media ads and wishful thinking, it's no wonder so many of us turn to little pots of pills and powders hoping they'll help us look, feel or function a little better.

So which ones are actually worth it?

Here's a quick guide to the best science-backed supplements for women to take during perimenopause – to support everything from muscle strength and cognitive performance to mood, immunity and sleep. And the good news? They aren't just for her – you'll benefit, too.

Discover more supplements that actually deliver at burningup-frozenout.com.

Ashwagandha

What? An adaptogenic herb that helps you handle pressure like the Dalai Lama.

Why? It lowers cortisol[102] (the main stress hormone) to ease anxiety, while also supporting memory and cognitive function.[103]

Pros: If reducing stress, sleeping better[104] and boosting brain power weren't enough, it may also increase strength gains and speed up recovery.[105]

Cons: It can lower blood pressure and blood sugar – a plus for some, a problem for others – and may interfere with certain medications, so check with your doctor first.[106]

Calcium

What? The bone-building mineral that also keeps muscles firing.

Why? Calcium maintains bone density to reduce the risk of osteoporosis. It's also involved in muscle function, nerve signalling and heart health.[107]

Pros: It strengthens bones and supports muscle and heart health so you can stay fit, strong and active as you age.

Cons: Too much calcium can increase the risk of kidney stones or heart issues, so stick to label guidelines.[108]

Creatine 101

The super supplement with serious benefits

If there's one supplement every woman should be taking in midlife, it's creatine.[109] Backed by decades of research, it delivers powerful physical and mental benefits in one safe, affordable and easy-to-take scoop.[110] From strength and stamina to sharper thinking and faster recovery, creatine is the ultimate all-rounder, and it works just as well for men, too. Here's what you need to know, from nutritional therapist, consultant and best-selling author Ian Marber (ianmarber.com).[111]

What is creatine?

Creatine is a compound found in red meat and fish, with many health and performance benefits. It fuels muscles to help them lift heavier and recover faster, supports energy levels, maintains bone density, and even sharpens memory and mental processing. Think of it as a cheat code for greater physical strength and better cognitive function.

Why do women need creatine?

Women store far less creatine in their bodies than men – up to 80 percent less[112] – primarily because it's stored in muscle tissue, and women typically have less muscle mass. Creatine is one of the best-researched, safest and most effective supplements for boosting muscle strength, athletic performance and brain power in both women and men. And if you're vegan or vegetarian, supplementation is especially important, since plant-based foods don't contain creatine.[113]

What does creatine do?

- Preserves muscle mass: it helps counteract age-related muscle loss (sarcopenia), which accelerates as hormone levels fall[114]
- Improves strength and performance: it enhances muscle function, making exercise more effective and enjoyable[115]
- Boosts brain function: it improves memory and focus to lift brain fog and combat long-term cognitive decline[116]
- Increases energy: it boosts cellular energy production to increase stamina and reduce fatigue[117]
- Supports bone health: it may help maintain and increase bone density to reduce the risk of osteoporosis[118]
- Aids recovery and reduces inflammation: it helps the body recover faster from exercise and everyday stress[119]

When should you take creatine?

Take creatine daily – timing matters less than consistency.[120] Some people prefer to take it after a workout because this may slightly enhance its uptake, but research shows it's equally effective before or at a completely different time of day.[121] The best option? Take it at the same time each day so it becomes routine. You can take it with or without food, though pairing it with carbs may improve absorption. Always drink water with it: creatine draws water into muscle cells, so staying hydrated maximizes its effects.[122]

How much creatine should you take?

Creatine monohydrate is the best (and cheapest) form and widely available.[123] The recommended daily dose is 3–5g.[124] There's no need for the 'loading' phase popularized by bodybuilders – consistent daily intake will eventually saturate muscle cells and deliver all the benefits.

Are there any side effects?

Creatine supplementation can cause digestive discomfort, and up to 30 percent of people may be 'non-responders', but for most people the benefits far outweigh any potential downsides.

Curcumin

What? The active compound in turmeric that delivers powerful anti-inflammatory benefits.

Why? Curcumin may help ease joint pain and reduce chronic inflammation throughout the body – a key driver of many age-related diseases.[125]

Pros: It's been shown to lower inflammation, protect cells from oxidative stress, and reduce the risk of long-term health conditions.[126]

Cons: Curcumin is poorly absorbed on its own,[127] so look for supplements that include black pepper extract (piperine) to boost its effectiveness.[128]

Vitamin D

What? An essential nutrient made by your skin when exposed to sunlight – and vital for many biological processes.[129]

Why? It supports calcium absorption to keep bones strong, strengthens the immune system to fight off illness, and may reduce the risk of chronic conditions like heart disease, diabetes and certain cancers.[130]

Pros: It's vital for long-term health, boosts energy, supports muscle function, and may lift mood, making it especially important as we age.[131]

Cons: It's hard to get enough from food alone, and if you don't get regular sun exposure – particularly in winter – you're likely deficient. Supplementation is a smart move.[132] For best absorption, take it with a source of dietary fat.

Magnesium

What? A multitasking mineral that's involved in more than 300 bodily functions.[133] It's found in leafy greens, nuts, seeds and wholegrains. Magnesium citrate and glycinate are the best supplemental forms.[134]

Why? Magnesium is essential for everyone, but especially important during perimenopause. It helps regulate oestrogen and progesterone to reduce mood swings, irritability and stress.[135] It also relaxes the nervous system to improve sleep onset and quality,[136] eases hot flushes and night sweats,[137] and keeps bones strong.[138]

Pros: In short, it's a midlife must-have for greater relaxation, recovery and resilience.

Cons: Some forms (like magnesium oxide) aren't well absorbed,[139] and too much can upset your stomach.[140] Start low and increase gradually to avoid any sudden bathroom sprints.

Protein powder

What? A powdered source of protein made from milk (whey and casein), eggs, soy, peas, rice, collagen or hemp. They're not just for bodybuilders, but for anyone wanting to boost their protein intake.

Why? Protein maintains muscle, supports metabolism, protects bones and more. Powders offer a quick and convenient way to top up daily intake.[141]

Pros: They deliver up to 30g of protein in one easy hit. Mix with milk or water for a shake, blend into a smoothie, or stir into porridge or yoghurt.

Cons: They should supplement, not replace, real food. Some are packed with sugar, sweeteners or fillers and may cause bloating.[142] Plant-based blends may lack all the essential amino acids.[143]

Omega-3 fatty acids

What? Omega-3s are essential fatty acids that your body can't produce on its own, so you have to get them from food or supplements.[144] There are three main types: EPA and DHA (found in oily fish like salmon and mackerel), and ALA (found in nuts and seeds).

Why? Omega-3s lower inflammation,[145] improve cholesterol[146] and reduce the risk of heart disease.[147] They also support brain function[148] and can reduce stiffness to make movement easier.[149]

Pros: They can improve heart health, help brain function and ease joint pain.

Cons: Fish burps are real. Taking omega-3s with food can help stop them repeating on you.

Rhodiola rosea

What? A stress-busting adaptogenic herb that helps you stay sharp, resilient and energized under pressure.

Why? It supports the body's stress response,[150] reduces mental and physical exhaustion,[151] and may improve mood and focus.[152] By balancing neurotransmitters like serotonin and dopamine, it helps you feel mentally clear and emotionally steady – without the jitters or crashes that come with caffeine.

Pros: It fights fatigue, boosts brain power and lifts mood – a natural pick-me-up for busy, stressed-out people.

Cons: It's mildly stimulating, so taking it too late in the day may interfere with sleep.[153]

From food to fitness

Smart food choices lay the foundation. The right supplements fill the gaps. But to thrive through perimenopause and beyond, there's one final piece of the puzzle: movement.

Exercise is what transforms potential into power and doubt into strength. It's not just about building muscle or blitzing belly fat – it boosts energy, clears brain fog, calms anxiety, and floods her body with feel-good hormones.

So no, it won't just change how she looks, it will rebuild her confidence, deepen her resilience and lift her sense of self-worth. And just like with food, this isn't about perfection. It's about progress. That's what the next chapter is about: helping her move more, move better – and feel unstoppable.

11

Move more
Exercise for strength, sanity and self-esteem

When everything feels off – energy, mood, sleep, body confidence – exercise is often the last thing on anyone's mind. Yet it's one of the most powerful ways to feel better ... and fast. Not because it burns calories but because it builds momentum. It sharpens her brain, lifts her mood, strengthens her bones, maintains her muscles, protects her heart and helps her sleep. It reconnects her with her body at a time when everything feels like it's falling apart. And it's the final cog in the virtuous cycle – once she starts moving, everything else becomes easier.

And here's the truth: it's not laziness that stops most women moving more. It's life. No time. No energy. No confidence. No idea where to start.

This chapter tackles all of it and gives you the tools, motivation and understanding to help her break through the barriers. Because once she starts, the benefits don't just show up in the mirror – they show up in her mind, her mood, your relationship and the future you're building together.

In this chapter you'll discover:
- Why exercise is the closest thing to a menopause 'cure'
- How lifting weights builds stronger bones, muscles and resilience
- The best types of cardio to clear brain fog, fight belly fat and beat anxiety
- The real reasons women don't exercise and how you can help
- How to rebuild momentum when motivation's gone missing
- What to do if she's scared, stuck or secretly hates exercise
- The weekly workout plan that works for beginners and pros alike
- Why training together builds confidence, connection and consistency.

Lifestyle lifeline #4: Move more

The most powerful thing she can do for her body and mind? Exercise.

Not detox diets. Not overpriced supplements. Not wishful thinking. Just regular, structured exercise. It's as close to a perimenopause panacea as you'll find.[1]

Why? Because when women stop moving, everything starts to slip.[2] Muscle mass declines. Bone density drops. Heart health suffers. Energy, mood and sleep all take a hit. Fat accumulates – especially around the middle – and with it comes a soaring risk of type-2 diabetes,[3] heart disease[4] and some cancers.[5]

Benefits for both of you

And it's not just her. Midlife is just as unforgiving for men who don't move. Sit still long enough and the effects soon show: weaker muscles, a softer waistline, rising blood pressure, fading stamina and a sex drive that's vanished without a trace.

That's why exercise isn't just a good idea at this life stage – it's essential. It's the one lifestyle habit with the power to improve every part of her physical and mental wellbeing, from body composition and brain function to mood, memory and motivation.

And the benefits don't stop there. Moving more – and moving better – isn't just about how she looks. It's about how she lives. Exercise builds resilience, boosts confidence, and restores a sense of control at a time of life when everything else can feel up in the air.[6]

But there's a problem.

It's not laziness – it's life

Most of us simply aren't moving enough.

Nearly four in ten women aged 45–54 don't hit the recommended target of 150 minutes of exercise per week.[7] And almost one in four are classed as 'physically inactive' – meaning they get less than 30 minutes a week, according to Sport England.[8]

The numbers aren't much better for men. Only 31 percent of middle-aged men reach the weekly 150-minute target.

If you ask her why she doesn't exercise as much as she'd like – or at all – chances are her answer will fall into one of the following categories.[9] And you'll probably recognize them from your own experience, too:

- **No time:** life's already a juggling act.
- **No energy:** she's running on empty.
- **No confidence:** the gym is intimidating.
- **No clue:** she doesn't know where to start.
- **No motivation:** exercise feels like yet another chore.
- **No space for self-care:** everyone else should come first.

Movement is medicine

These aren't excuses – they're real obstacles. And with three in ten women becoming less active during menopause, the barriers need breaking down.[10] (The second half of this chapter is packed with practical ways to do exactly that, and they'll work for you, too.)

Why? Because regular exercise can significantly reduce many of the toughest perimenopause symptoms,[11] including brain fog,[12] fatigue,[13] hot flushes[14] and weight gain.[15] It also improves long-term health outcomes dramatically.[16]

How? Many of the leading causes of death in women are all linked to falling oestrogen, which usually offers protection against heart disease, obesity and type-2 diabetes, as well as muscle loss, brittle bones (hip fractures are strongly associated with increased mortality in older women) and even dementia.

Regular exercise can offset the loss of oestrogen's protective effects by:

- improving heart health and lowering blood pressure[17]
- increasing insulin sensitivity to reduce the risk of obesity and type-2 diabetes[18]
- building muscle mass size and strength[19]
- improving coordination and balance[20]
- maintaining bone density to reduce risk and severity of fall-related injuries[21]
- boosting cognitive function and supporting long-term brain health.[22]

And that's the point: exercise isn't just about losing weight or feeling a bit fitter. Without it, we lose health, confidence and independence with every passing year.

Everything she's been told about exercise is wrong

As if low energy, zero time and no confidence weren't enough, she's also been misled by two exercise myths so widespread they're practically gospel.

The first? That lifting anything heavier than a handbag would turn even Dame Judi Dench into Dwayne 'The Rock' Johnson. (Men know that's nonsense – many of us have spent years lifting weights, yet look more suited to sumo wrestling than the WWE.)

The second? That the only way to burn fat is endless, slow, boring cardio. In fact, lifting weights and short bursts of intense cardio are far more effective and take far less time.[23] We'll explain how shortly.

The myths that kill motivation

These misconceptions have kept even the most motivated women out of the weights room and stuck in the safe zone of gentle cardio or yoga. While those types of training are great for heart health and flexibility, they don't deliver the muscle-strengthening or bone-building benefits of lifting weights – the kind that unlock a longer, stronger, more independent life.

And that matters. Remember, two of the biggest long-term health risks for women are rapid muscle loss (and the strength that goes with it) and declining bone density. In short: they become weaker, more fragile and far less capable of living life on their own terms.

Strong is the new skinny

So, what kind of exercise is best?

Lifting weights. And heavy ones – not those dainty pink dumbbells that would struggle as a paperweight.

Strength training – which involves using your muscles to push, pull or lift against resistance (from dumbbells, barbells, resistance bands, machines, or even your own bodyweight) – is the best way to build strength, protect bones and support metabolism as we age.[24]

It also helps counter the hormonal chaos of midlife,[25] especially the drop in oestrogen that accelerates muscle loss, weakens bones and makes it easier to store fat. Lifting weights fights back against all of it. Every rep is an act of rebellion against ageing.

As leading female exercise physiologist Dr Stacy Sims puts it: 'Strength training is what keeps women out of a nursing home.'

The same is true for you. And once you know what to do, you'll have the power to transform not just your own life – but hers, too.

The four training types that matter most

The four most important forms of exercise in midlife – and at any age – are:

- **Strength training**[26]
- **High-intensity interval training (HIIT)**[27]
- **Plyometric training**[28]
- **Low-intensity steady-state (LISS) cardio.**[29]

We'll get into each specific type shortly, but here's the top line, according to Dr Sims.

Strength training is the most important and should be prioritized above everything else. Then comes **HIIT** – short bursts of all-out effort, like sprinting, between longer recovery periods. **Plyometric training** involves explosive moves like box jumps and squat jumps. Then there's **low-intensity steady-state cardio** (LISS, for short – unless you like tongue-twisters) – jogging, cycling, hiking, swimming – the stuff most people visualize when they think of 'exercise'. The simplest way to think about it? Each training type plays a unique and essential role in supporting physical health and mental wellbeing, and a smart combination of all four delivers the best results – reducing perimenopause symptoms (for her) and improving long-term health (for both of you).

The Exercise Priority Pyramid

Meet the Exercise Priority Pyramid – an easy guide to fitting the different training types together into a weekly plan.

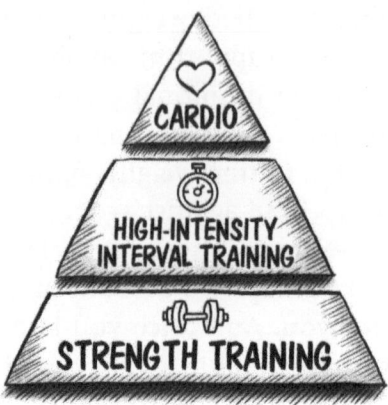

At the base is strength training – the foundation of fitness, health and independence. Above that is HIIT – which improves heart, lung and brain function while torching calories and boosting metabolic health. On top sits LISS – ideal for recovery, building endurance, reducing stress and lifting mood.[30] Plyometric training – short, sharp bursts of jumping or explosive movement – can be added to the start or end of strength or HIIT sessions to boost explosive power, balance and coordination.

Sounds like a lot? Don't sweat it: there are plenty of smart, time-saving ways to get it done – even with a packed schedule – and we're going to show you how.

She's not just lifting weights – she's learning to believe in herself

Before we get into why each type of training is so powerful – and how to do it – let's consider how women approach exercise, especially strength training. Pumping iron might feel second nature to you – straightforward, instinctive. You may even own a pair of dumbbells (even if they only get lifted when you move house). But for many women, it's a completely different story.

Overcoming the fear factor

On the surface, strength training sounds simple: pick up something heavy, put it down, repeat.

But dig a little deeper and it's a seismic shift. Because this isn't just about exercise – it's about questioning a deeply ingrained inner narrative:[31] one that says what she enjoys, what her body can do, and what kind of person she is or could become.

And it's not just lifting. The same goes for certain types of cardio, too. You've probably done your fair share of running or five-a-side football, so a HIIT workout feels doable. But if she's never done it before – or always thought sprint training was just for professional athletes – even the thought can feel intimidating.[32]

That's why baby steps matter. Not just to avoid injury or get better results but to make sure training feels good from the start, so it becomes something she wants to do, not something she feels she has to do.

And speaking of making training safe, effective and enjoyable, there's one more thing you need to know. It's something a lot of women still get wrong ...

Should women train on an empty stomach?

In a word: no.[33]

A lot of people think working out on an empty stomach – aka fasted training – is a short cut to fat-loss success. It sounds logical: skip breakfast, burn calories, force the body to tap into fat stores for fuel. Right?

Wrong. At least, not when it comes to women.[34] In fact, it's one of the worst things she can do.

Fasted training can work for men because their bodies are biologically built to handle that kind of energy deficit. But, for women, it's a different story. When she trains without fuel, her body panics and switches into calorie-saving mode. Instead of burning fat, it starts breaking down muscle for energy.

This was a useful survival mechanism in our hunter-gatherer past,[35] but today it's a fast-track to burnout. Doing high-intensity or strength workouts fasted can leave her feeling drained and sluggish during the session and depleted afterwards – all while eating away at the muscle she's trying to build. But, according to Dr Sims, there's a simple fix ... and it's delicious.

Strength sessions: Before a weights workout, she should consume around 15g of protein – that's a couple of boiled eggs, a small serving of Greek yoghurt, or a protein coffee. (To make the protein coffee, mix 15g of protein powder with 120ml, or 4 fl. oz, of cold milk, stir until smooth, then add a double shot, or 60ml/2 fl. oz, of cold coffee. Store it in the fridge overnight if prepping ahead.)

This signals to her body that nutrition is on the way, helping to preserve muscle and keep her metabolism firing. Don't stress about the calories: there are only about 60 in 15g of protein, and she'll burn far more in the next 48 hours thanks to the post-workout metabolic boost. Follow up with a high-protein meal to support muscle repair and growth.

Cardio workouts: She should aim for 15g of protein and 30g of carbs – think a couple of eggs on toast, or a small bowl of Greek yoghurt with fruit and honey. This adds up to just under 200 calories, enough to fuel her session and protect muscle tissue. As with strength training, a high-protein meal afterwards will speed up recovery and improve results.

Activewear 101

The clothes that boost confidence and performance

One last thing before we get to the training itself, and it's a big one. You might be perfectly happy training in a faded pair of football shorts and a Radiohead tour T-shirt from 1997, but what she wears for her workouts isn't just a fashion statement – it can make or break the session.

The right clothes not only support performance (no sports bra = no running or jumping), but also, more importantly, boost confidence. If she feels good in what she's wearing, she's far more likely to show up, push herself and enjoy it. If she feels self-conscious? She might not even make it out of the changing room.[36]

What's more, plenty of brands now offer wallet-friendly ranges that tick both the comfort and performance boxes, so you won't need to sell a kidney to kit her out in Sweaty Betty. Here's what every woman's workout wardrobe needs.

Sports bra

A good sports bra provides essential support and protects breast tissue during high-impact movement. Without one, running or jumping becomes awkward and painful. Bras with wide straps, moisture-wicking fabric, and a snug fit that doesn't dig in are best, and steer clear of fashion-first options that prioritize style over structure.

Leggings

They might all look the same to you, but trust us, not all leggings are created equal. She'll want a pair that are breathable, sweat-wicking, high-waisted (so she's not hitching them up every two minutes) and squat-proof – meaning they won't turn see-through the second she bends over (behave). Four-way stretch is a must so she can move freely, and avoid anything thin, low-rise or made from cotton – unless she's going for the saggy, sweaty look (she's not).

Tops

Tops should be comfortable, breathable and suited to the intensity of her workout. Sleeveless styles offer maximum freedom to move and help keep things cool, but some women prefer to keep their arms covered. Same goes for fit: not so tight it shrink-wraps her belly, not so loose it rides up mid-burpee. The sweet spot? Lightweight tops made from technical fabric, with a longer cut and a bit of shape. Avoid thick cotton that traps heat and sweat, or anything that needs constant adjusting – keeping herself covered shouldn't be part of the workout.

Trainers

The right shoes depend on the type of workout. Running shoes should offer good cushioning, arch support, and shock absorption – and it's worth getting a gait analysis at a specialist shop before splashing the cash, so she gets the right support for her stride. For strength training or HIIT, stability matters more than cushioning, so flat, grippy soles are the better option.

The four training types explained

Now she's fuelled up and kitted out, it's time to break down the four types of exercise that matter most. Each one plays a different role – from building strength to boosting stamina – and together, they create the ultimate feel-good formula.

Training type #1: Strength training

> AKA lifting heavy things
> Key benefits: Builds and maintains muscle and bone
> Key moves: Squats, deadlifts, presses, rows

What? Strength training involves using your muscles to lift and lower heavy things. The most common equipment includes barbells, dumbbells, machines or your own bodyweight. The best exercises are compound lifts: squats, deadlifts, lunges, bench presses, overhead presses, bent-over rows and lat pulldowns (see below).

Why? 'If women are only going to do one thing, it should be strength training,' says renowned exercise physiologist Dr Stacy Sims. Falling oestrogen levels cause muscle and bone loss, slow down metabolism, and make it easier to store fat and harder to lose it. Lifting weights fights back against all of it – and more – to massively boost long-term health. It's just as vital for men, too: strength training builds muscle and mental resilience, burns fat, boosts testosterone (and libido), and improves overall health.

When? Dr Sims recommends women strength train three times a week: one session focused on lower-body moves (think squats and lunges), one on upper-body moves (like shoulder presses and rows), and one on posterior chain moves (exercises for the back of the body, like deadlifts and hip thrusts). If time's tight, two full-body sessions a week will do the job – just make sure they include squats, deadlifts and a pressing and pulling move for the upper body.

Strength training 101

The non-negotiable foundation of fitness

It's not about bulking up. It's about building back what perimenopause tries to take away – strength, stability, energy, focus and confidence. Here's why lifting heavy might just be the most powerful move she'll ever make.

It stops her getting weaker, wobblier and worn out

Another of oestrogen's many roles is aiding muscle repair.[37] So, when it drops, muscles shrink and weaken – known as sarcopenia[38] – and everyday tasks become harder. But strength training fights back. It creates tiny tears in muscle fibres that grow back bigger and stronger – when paired with enough protein. The payoff? More muscle, greater strength and better balance and coordination to make life that much easier again.[39]

It builds bones that won't break

Fragile bones are a big problem. In the UK, around 3.5 million people have osteoporosis, and one in two women over 50 will suffer a fracture.[40] That's because, during the five to seven years after menopause, women can lose up to 20 percent of their bone mass.[41] In fact, a woman's risk of breaking her hip is the same as her combined risk of breast, uterine and ovarian cancer.[42] Strength training can stop the decline by putting healthy stress on bones and joints, making them stronger and more resilient.[43] It also helps prevent painful perimenopausal injuries like frozen shoulder and plantar fasciitis that make movement a misery.[44]

It burns belly fat – and keeps it off

Strength training is one of the quickest ways to shed excess belly fat – and keep it off – boosting body confidence at a time when she's struggling to accept her changing shape.[45] But a muffin top isn't just upsetting – it's a flashing warning sign. Strength training improves insulin sensitivity, helping the body manage blood sugar better, which reduces weight gain and cuts the long-term risk of type-2 diabetes.[46] And thanks to its after-burn effect (aka excess post-exercise oxygen consumption, or EPOC), her body keeps burning extra calories for hours after a workout.[47]

It clears brain fog and boosts her mood

Lifting heavy things triggers the release of brain-derived neurotrophic factor (BDNF),[48] often described as Miracle-Gro for the brain, which boosts cognitive function, memory and mood.[49] Add a wave of feel-good endorphins that combat anxiety – and suddenly the world feels more manageable.[50] The best bit? Many women experience more energy and better sleep within weeks of getting started.[51]

It gives her power, pride and purpose

Yes, she'll get stronger, leaner and have more energy. But one of the biggest benefits? Feeling like a total badass.[52] Strength training isn't just about lifting weights – it's about realizing what she's capable of. By taking the fight to Father Time she's refusing to let her confidence or resilience slip away. Being able to handle whatever life throws at her builds the kind of self-belief nothing else can touch.

The four big power moves

These are the foundational lifts that should form the backbone of every strength workout. They work multiple muscle groups at once, build strength faster and deliver bigger results. Get more moves and form guides at burningupfrozenout.com.

Power move #1: Squat

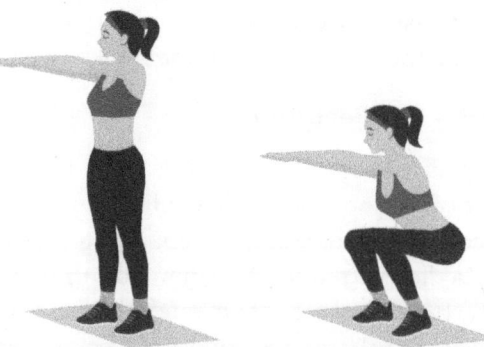

Muscles worked: Quads and hamstrings (thighs), glutes (bum), core (abs and lower back). Also improves balance, coordination and overall mobility.

How to do it: Stand tall with feet shoulder-width apart and arms straight out in front. Keep the chin and chest up with a straight back. Bend the knees and push the bum backward to squat down – as if sitting into a chair – until the thighs are parallel to the floor. Drive back up through the heels to stand back up.

Beginner's tip: Start with bodyweight squats to master the form and build confidence. Then add resistance with dumbbells, kettlebells or a barbell.

Power move #2: Straight-leg deadlift

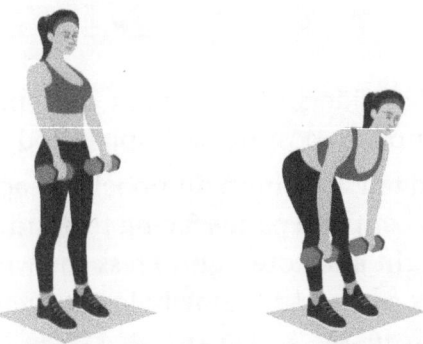

Muscles worked: Hamstrings, glutes and lower back (AKA the posterior chain). Also improves your ability to lift and lower things safely – an essential life skill.

How to do it: Stand tall with feet hip-width apart, holding a dumbbell in each hand with an overhand grip in front of the thighs. With the chin up and back straight, bend forward from the hips to lower the weights towards the floor until there's a good stretch in the backs of your thighs. Then reverse the movement to return to the start.

Beginner's tip: Start with no weights. Place your hands on your thighs and slide them down your legs as you hinge at the hips, keeping your back flat. Stop when you feel the stretch in your hamstrings, then return to standing. Once that feels natural, add light dumbbells or a kettlebell.

Power move #3: Shoulder press

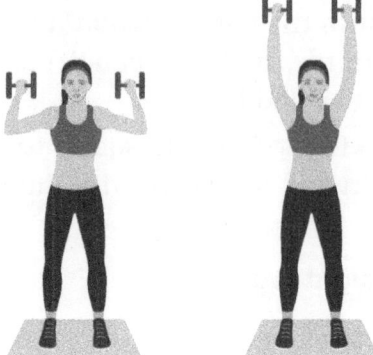

Muscles worked: Shoulders, triceps (back of upper arms) and upper chest. Also helps improve posture and upper-body strength.

How to do it: Stand tall, holding a dumbbell in each hand at shoulder height with elbows bent and palms facing forward. Keep the chin and chest up, back straight and core tight. Press the weights directly overhead until the arms are straight. Slowly lower them back to the start.

Beginner's tip: Use light dumbbells or resistance bands to build strength and control. Gradually increase the weight as you get stronger.

Power move #4: Bent-over row

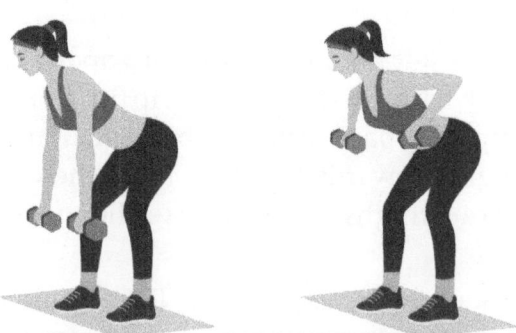

Muscles worked: Upper and lower back, rear shoulders and core. Also helps undo the slouched posture that comes from too much desk time.

How to do it: Stand tall with a dumbbell in each hand or both hands holding a barbell. With back straight, knees slightly bent and core tight, lean forward. Row the weight up until the hands are either side of the torso, squeezing the shoulder blades together at the top. Reverse the movement to return to the start.

Beginner's tip: Imagine balancing a broomstick along your spine – your head, back and hips should stay aligned throughout the move.

Instant expert

Dr Stacy Sims on helping her fall in love with lifting

Dr Stacy Sims is a world-leading exercise physiologist and nutrition scientist whose game-changing research and books on female physiology have redefined how women should train.[53] Here's how you can be the supportive partner she needs – not just to start lifting weights, but to fall in love with the strength, confidence and control it gives her (drstacysims.com).

Start where she's at, not where she wants to be

Heavy deadlifts and overhead squats aren't day-one moves. If she's new to strength training – or hasn't done any structured exercise in years – the key is to start gently and progress gradually. Help her embrace the idea that Rome wasn't built in a day. Simple bodyweight moves like air squats, walking lunges or wall push-ups will build both strength and confidence. In time, invest in some dumbbells or kettlebells for tougher home workouts, or help her find a beginner-friendly gym or personal trainer.

Make it about feeling strong, powerful and confident, not looking slimmer

One of the fastest wins from lifting weights isn't visible – it's felt. Within a few weeks of strength training, many women notice better balance, deeper sleep, less joint pain, more energy and sharper thinking. So, although she might not see a change in the mirror immediately, her body is changing in all the right ways. Be the one who notices she's walking taller, sleeping better or seems more confident. Celebrate those shifts proudly and remind her lifting weights isn't about punishment or perfection – it's about power.

Empower her to lift well, not just lift heavy

When she's starting out, good form matters more than big weights. Remind her it's a journey – building to a heavy lift can take a year or more, and that's perfectly normal. Learning to move well before loading up is the key to real strength, and injury prevention, especially with hormonal changes increasing the risk of issues like frozen shoulder or plantar fasciitis. Offer to film her so she can check her form, but don't become her coach. Your role is to be her cheerleader, not her drill sergeant. Leave that to a personal trainer who's getting paid to put up with the potty mouth and death stares.

Give her the time and space to train

If she wants to train with you – brilliant. Your presence can make weight rooms feel less intimidating, and your experience might help fast-track her progress. But if she'd rather lift solo or with a female friend, step aside – and step up elsewhere. Women often feel guilty prioritizing their own fitness, especially while juggling everything else. So lighten the load elsewhere to give her the time – and headspace – to train. Make sure that time is protected, respected and celebrated. It might feel like a chore now, but you'll both reap the rewards in the long run.

Remind her she's building a better future

Strength training in midlife isn't a luxury – it's a long-term investment. Every squat, press and row is a down payment on decades of strength, confidence and independence. And the best part? It's never too late to start – but the sooner she does, the stronger her future will be.

Train for today – and for tomorrow

Struggling to find motivation today? Think of the long game. A few minutes of movement now can protect your future self. Three of the strongest predictors of long-term health and lifespan? Muscle strength, lean muscle mass and VO_2 max.[54] Train for them – and for the decades to come.

Home gym essentials: Get strong without going out

Forget what Instagram shows you. She doesn't need a fancy gym membership or a sleek home gym packed with expensive kit to get fitter and stronger. All she needs to get started is a pair of heavy(ish) dumbbells.

As she gets stronger, a few extra bits of kit will help her progress and add variety. But building a home gym doesn't mean blowing the budget. Here's what to buy first – and why – according to women's fitness coach Kate Rowe-Ham (owningyourmenopause.com).

1 Dumbbells: The must-have muscle builder

If there's only room (or budget) for one bit of kit, make it dumbbells. They're versatile, beginner-friendly, and brilliant for strengthening every major muscle group.

A medium pair (6–8kg) works well for lower-body moves like squats, lunges and deadlifts, and upper-body push–pull moves for the chest and back.

If she can stretch to three pairs, even better:

- Light (2–4kg) for shoulders and arms
- Medium (6–8kg) for chest and back
- Heavy (10kg+) for legs and glutes.

Short on space? Adjustable dumbbells are a smart space-saving option – offering a range of weights in one set – but they're not cheap.

2 Resistance bands: A secret weapon for strength and stability

Resistance bands are cheap and cheerful but very challenging. They can warm up muscles before a session and stretch them afterwards, and can add extra resistance to bodyweight and dumbbell lifts. Use light bands for upper-body moves, medium bands for mobility and core work, and heavier ones for lower-body lifts.

3 A bench or step: Add variety and unlock power

A bench opens up a whole new range of bodyweight, dumbbell and barbell moves, such as dips, bench presses and step-ups. If space or money is tight, an aerobic-style step with adjustable height is a good option.

4 Kettlebells: For strength moves to sweaty sessions

A kettlebell might look like an oversized doorstop, but it's a seriously effective bit of strength-training kit and great for HIIT-style workouts, too. She can use it for classic strength moves like squats, deadlifts, lunges, presses and rows, or dial things up with fast-paced circuits featuring swings, cleans and snatches. These dynamic exercises raise the heart rate, work the core to stabilize the body, and improve balance, timing and coordination. A moderate-weight kettlebell (8–12kg) is a solid place to start.

5 Mat and mirror: Get extra comfort, support and feedback

A good exercise mat makes floor work, for core and mobility moves as well as stretching, far more comfortable and helps prevent slipping. And while a mirror might sound like a vanity purchase it's actually a great tool for checking form and making sure she's moving correctly. It builds confidence, reduces the risk of injury and offers instant visual feedback, which is especially useful when training alone at home.

Training type #2: High-intensity interval training

> AKA Moving freaking fast
> Key benefits: Improves heart health and reduces belly fat
> Key moves: Kettlebell swings, sprints, circuit training

What? HIIT involves short bursts of near-maximal effort followed by longer periods of rest. Think 30 seconds of kettlebell swings, battle ropes or running sprints, followed by a couple of minutes of recovery, repeated for a few rounds. It's fast, brutal and efficient – a HIIT session can be done in less than 20 minutes – but it delivers.

Why? 'Research shows that HIIT helps preserve lean muscle mass and help recruit our powerful fast-twitch muscle fibres, which we want to maintain as we age,' says Dr Alyssa Olenick, an exercise physiologist specializing in female physiology. HIIT is also one of the most effective ways to boost insulin sensitivity, improve cardiovascular fitness and counteract the metabolic dysregulation many women face during perimenopause.

When? Once the strength training is in place, aim for one or two short HIIT sessions each week, with a focus on quality over quantity. That means going hard enough during the 'work' periods with sufficient 'rest' periods between them. But, as Dr Olenick warns, HIIT can be incredibly physically and mentally taxing, especially if you're new to it. That makes circuit-style intervals or stationary bike sprints a better bet than all-out running sprints.

Cardio 101

Critical for hormones, heart health and headspace

Cardio isn't just about burning calories: it's essential for heart and lung health, better brain function and mental wellbeing, and much more. Here's how everything from intense intervals to relaxed countryside walks can help counteract many of the most disruptive symptoms caused by falling hormone levels.

Strengthen her heart, save her life

Oestrogen protects the heart, so when levels drop the risk of cardiovascular disease (CVD) rises.[55] In the UK, CVD causes almost one in five of all female deaths in the 55 to 74 age group, and 2.8 million women currently live with the disease.[56] Regular cardio strengthens the heart, improves blood flow, lowers blood pressure and can significantly cut risk – especially if started during perimenopause.[57]

Burn belly fat, boost body confidence

Falling oestrogen flips where fat gets stored,[58] shifting it from the hips and thighs to the stomach, reshaping her body and rattling her confidence.[59] Cardio training can stop fat gain by burning existing fat stores, improving insulin sensitivity and supporting overall energy balance and metabolic health.[60]

Reset her mood and mind

Cardio triggers a rush of endorphins that can fight back against mood swings and emotional crashes. So if it all gets too much – when energy, mood and motivation are at rock bottom – there's nothing better than getting into nature and moving. Just 20 minutes of walking can lower stress hormone levels by more than 20 percent.[61] Cardio also reduces anxiety and improves sleep, which builds even greater resilience.[62]

Build grit that lasts for life

Cardio isn't just good for the heart – it's also great for the head.[63] Whether it's grinding out the final 30 seconds of a sprint or pushing through the last set of kettlebell swings, cardio teaches us how to tolerate (and maybe even embrace) short spells of discomfort. That grit builds mental toughness, confidence and self-belief – skills that spill over into every other part of life.[64]

Move to reconnect and recharge

Not all cardio has to be fast or furious. Often, it's the slow and steady stuff – a long walk, a gentle swim, or a ride through the countryside – that feeds the soul and makes the world a better place.[65] Done solo, it can be a quiet sanctuary from everyday chaos. Done with friends or family, it can be a powerful way to connect, reflect and deepen supportive relationships.[66] In short, cardio helps her reconnect with herself and the people who matter most.[67]

Training type #3: Low-intensity steady-state (LISS) cardio

> AKA movement for mind and soul
> Key benefits: Reduces stress, improves sleep, promotes recovery
> Key activities: Jogging, hiking, swimming, cycling

What? LISS is all about moving at a steady, easy pace. It's the kind of cardio during which you can comfortably chat without gasping for air. Steady-state cardio might not be the main priority, but it's still essential – especially for mental wellbeing.

Why? 'LISS training is really underrated because many people view it as too easy to be effective,' says Dr Olenick. 'But walking, cycling or swimming can support fat loss, improve sleep, and is a valuable form of active recovery to complement weight lifting and more intense forms of cardio.' It's also a brilliant way to decompress – whether she's catching up with someone or simply taking a break from the noise. Most importantly, it's often the only kind of movement that feels doable on low-energy days, when the alternative is doing nothing.

When? As often as possible. Low-intensity movement can be done on rest days, after strength or HIIT sessions, or whenever energy is low. It doesn't require a strict plan – just movement. The rough goal should be a heart rate between 50 and 70 percent of your max for around 20–30 minutes, but as little as 10 minutes is fine. Think of LISS less as a workout and more of a physical and mental reset – a pocket of calm on even the most chaotic days.

> ### Real talk
>
> **'Exercise helped me lose 100lb, but what I've gained is so much more'**
>
> *I'm Melanie. I'm 56, I live in Murphy, North Carolina, and I work as a real estate consultant.*
>
> There was a point – not too long ago – when I was approved for gastric bypass surgery. I'd tried everything. At my heaviest I was 280lb (127kg) – maybe more. I'd stopped weighing myself. I couldn't bear to see the number on the scale.
>
> But something in me said: Give it one more go. That was seven years ago. I started with boot camps, then I found Peloton and, eventually, strength training. Now I'm a competitive cyclist – after spending my whole life thinking being an athlete was something other people did.
>
> I've now lost over 100lb (45kg). But honestly? That's not what I'm most proud of. The real gain has been confidence. Strength. Independence. I've got two young grandkids and I can keep up with them no problem. I can open jars, carry shopping, and move through life feeling capable and in control.
>
> This is the first time in my life I can look in the mirror and feel proud of what I see – not because I look like a model, but because I built this body. I earned this strength. That's where real self-esteem comes from.
>
> Do I wish I'd started earlier? Absolutely. But I thank God I started when I did. It's never too late.
>
> If I could give one piece of advice to other women? Get through the gym door that first time. It's not as scary as it seems. Find something you enjoy – running, cycling, swimming. Ask for help if you need it. And keep showing up. You're stronger than you think.

Training type #4: Plyometrics

> AKA leaping like the floor is lava
> Key benefits: Builds power, protects bone, improves balance and coordination
> Key moves: Box jumps, jump squats, skipping

What? Plyometrics sound complicated but are actually very simple: they're just jumping-based movements – like hops, skips, and jumps – performed explosively to train the body to produce and absorb force quickly. This type of training improves speed, power and coordination, and strengthens muscles, bones and tendons to withstand impact more safely.

Why? 'Plyometrics are essential because they stimulate the muscle–nerve connection the way oestrogen used to,' says Dr Sims. 'This kind of impact work helps preserve bone density and improves muscle power and coordination – all of which decline rapidly during perimenopause.'

When? Plyometrics are best done once or twice per week as part of a warm-up before a strength session or HIIT workout, or as a 'finisher' – the final component of one of those sessions before cooling down. Women with joint issues or pelvic floor concerns should consult a physio or trainer before doing high-impact plyometrics. And even with a clean bill of health, it's best to start simple and safe with low-impact hops and skips to build confidence and give the body time to adjust.

Instant expert

Dr Alyssa Olenick on helping her train smarter, not harder

Dr Alyssa Olenick is an exercise physiologist, ultramarathon runner and hybrid coach who helps women make cardio work – without the grind, guilt or guesswork. Here's how you can help your partner ditch the dread, embrace movement, and finally find a routine she can stick to.

Make it fun, not furious

In desperation to lose weight, many women default to hours of high-intensity training. But cardio needs to be clever, and that means planning it to better balance harder and lower-effort sessions. Too much can leave her exhausted rather than energized – especially when hormonal changes prolong recovery and raise stress levels. If she's feeling run down, frustrated or not seeing results, encourage her to shift focus from punishing workouts to effective ones. Then support her by suggesting a bike ride together or a game of tennis or another sport she enjoys. By making exercise fun, you take the focus – and pressure – off obsessing over results.

Walk daily, win big

If exercise has been sidelined since school, it needs to be eased back in. Don't try to make up for lost time by doing too much too soon. A brisk walk may not sound like much, but is a better option than nothing when energy and motivation are too low for lifting weights or high-intensity training. As fitness improves, longer or hillier walks and hikes will become a pleasure rather than another chore.

Ride, run, dance, repeat

Running is a fantastic activity, but there are many other cardio options, especially for women new or returning to exercise. Support her in finding modes of movement she actually enjoys and can stick with. Whether it's cycling, swimming or dancing, the best form of cardio is the one she likes and wants to do again. Exercise should feel accessible, not intimidating. The goal is sustainability, not suffering.

Sweat together, stick together

Sticking to a new fitness kick is much easier when you're not doing it alone. Having you involved – whether that's keeping her company on a long walk, tagging along to a class, or swinging kettlebells when she rests (and vice versa) – can be the difference between a healthy habit lasting or falling at the first hurdle. Why? Accountability and camaraderie make it easier to get it done, especially when energy or motivation dips.

Ditch the guilt-trip workouts

If she doesn't want to train with you, don't take it personally. Encourage her to exercise with a friend or join a class. You can also help her reframe her mindset: many women still see exercise as a punishment for eating or drinking too much, rather than an essential act of self-care. Help her prioritize progress over perfection, and celebrate every win, no matter how small.

Putting a plan in place

You now know how the different types of training can improve everything from her muscle strength to her mood. But understanding the benefits of strength training, HIIT and cardio is one thing – without a plan, it's unlikely to stick.

That's why a weekly training programme matters. It ensures nothing gets missed, helps workouts complement rather than compete with each other, and builds in enough rest and variety to keep her body – and motivation – moving in the right direction. A plan also makes training feel more doable. No second-guessing. No decision fatigue. Just a clear roadmap that supports her goals, energy levels and busy life.

The sample weekly plans below show exactly how to make that happen – whatever her current fitness level.

> ### Short, sharp and sweaty
>
> These plans might look a little time-consuming on paper, but sessions don't have to be long. In fact, the most effective strength or HIIT workouts are often short and intense.
>
> Wherever she's beginning from, the golden rule is consistency. Training doesn't need to be perfect, but it does need to be regular. Progress slowly, make sure she listens to her body, and keep reminding her: the goal isn't just performance or aesthetics – it's strength, confidence and long-term health. You'll find programmes for all experience levels – for her and for you – at burningupfrozenout.com.

Beginner weekly plan

This suggested schedule for complete beginners includes two strength sessions: one for the lower body and one for the upper body. Strength workouts can start with bodyweight moves or light weights at home – the focus should be on good form before adding more resistance.

There's also one HIIT workout and one LISS activity, such as cycling, jogging or swimming. Walking can be done on rest days.

Monday	Strength training – lower body
Tuesday	Rest
Wednesday	HIIT session
Thursday	Strength training – upper body
Friday	Rest
Saturday	LISS cardio
Sunday	Rest

Intermediate weekly plan

This weekly outline is suited to those with recent experience of lifting weights or doing intense cardio. It features two strength sessions – one lower body and one upper body – plus an optional third total-body session that includes posterior-chain exercises like Romanian deadlifts, hip thrusts or glute bridges to build strength where many women are weakest: the hamstrings, glutes and lower back. There's also one HIIT session and one LISS activity. Plyometric exercises can be included before or after one or two of the strength sessions.

Monday	Strength training – lower body
Tuesday	Rest
Wednesday	HIIT
Thursday	Strength training – upper body
Friday	Rest
Saturday	Strength training – total body (optional)
Sunday	LISS cardio

Advanced weekly plan

This programme is ideal for highly experienced trainees with a strong foundation in weight training and HIIT. It includes three strength sessions, two HIIT workouts and one LISS activity. Add a couple of plyometric exercises at the beginning or end of one strength session and one HIIT workout, and include mobility or range-of-motion work into warm-ups and cool-downs to improve flexibility, joint health and injury prevention.

Monday	Strength training – lower body
Tuesday	Sprint training
Wednesday	Strength training – upper body
Thursday	Rest
Friday	Strength training – total body
Saturday	HIIT
Sunday	LISS cardio

The dirty dozen: Overcoming the top 12 exercise excuses

Even with all the knowledge, support and good intentions in the world, life gets in the way. These are the most common obstacles that stand between her and consistent training, and how you can remove them:

1. **'I don't have time.'** Between work, family and running a household, her to-do list is longer than Elton John's florist receipt.
   Fix it: Take something off her plate – do the food shop, hang up the laundry – anything that gives her some time to move, no strings, no stress.
2. **'I'm too tired.'** Perimenopausal fatigue is no joke. Some days, putting on a sports bra can feel like solving a Rubik's Cube in the dark with your hands tied behind your back (we've been told).
   Fix it: On low-energy days, suggest low-impact but re-energizing activities like walking, yoga or stretching that get her moving without requiring much brain power. And tag along on her stroll – before long, you'll have clocked more miles than the Proclaimers.
3. **'I feel self-conscious.'** Ever gone to a funeral in fancy dress? Everyone stares and wonders what the hell you're playing at. That's what walking into a gym for the first time feels like.
   Fix it: Help her find a female-friendly gym or a beginner-focused class or programme. Offer to go with her – or back off if she wants space. Do whatever builds confidence, not pressure.
4. **'I'm scared of leaking – or worse.'** It's not just a post-baby problem. Years – or even decades – after giving birth, worries about pelvic floor issues like leaking, discomfort, or prolapse can be a

real barrier to exercise. And it's not just mums: these concerns can affect anyone.

Fix it: Help her take things at her own pace. Start with low-impact, pelvic floor-friendly walking, swimming, yoga or bodyweight strength training with good form. If worries persist, encourage her to speak to a women's health physio – they can offer targeted exercises, reassurance and expert support.

5 **'I don't know what I'm doing.'** With every Instagram fitness influencer saying something different, it's no wonder she doesn't know her kettlebell swings from her split squats.

Fix it: Point her towards a simple, structured plan (get one for free at burningupfrozenout.com), or shout her a couple of sessions with a personal trainer who specializes in perimenopausal training.

6 **'It feels like another chore.'** If exercise seems like yet another box to tick, it'll slide down the priority list between colour-coding the sock drawer and alphabetizing the spice rack.

Fix it: Help her rediscover activities she used to love – like dancing, swimming or cycling. When movement feels like play and not punishment, it becomes a joy, not a chore.

7 **'I feel guilty prioritizing myself.'** She's been the family's unpaid chef, PA, therapist and crisis-response unit for years. No wonder taking time for herself feels extravagant.

Fix it: Tell her directly – and often – that she's allowed to put herself first. Exercise isn't something she has to earn. It's what helps her stay sane. That's not self-indulgent – that's a survival strategy.

8 **'I'm not seeing results.'** She's eating better and moving more, but her jeans haven't got the memo.

Fix it: Skip the scales and track the Midlife MOT wins that really matter more than her waistline – like greater energy, better sleep and happier moods.

9 **'I used to be fit, but I've lost it.'** She used to run 10km before breakfast, lift weights at lunch and dance all night, but now just putting on her trainers feels like a workout in itself.

Fix it: Don't let her get stuck comparing herself to her mid-twenties highlight reel. The goal isn't to beat her former self – it's to back her present one.

10 **'I must make up for lost time.'** She's ready to go full Rocky montage after years of inactivity, but going too hard too soon is as risky as doing nothing.
Fix it: Applaud the enthusiasm, but redirect the energy. This isn't about overnight transformation – it's about building momentum she can actually stick to. Slow and steady beats sore and sidelined.

11 **'I've tried before and failed.'** The drawer of never-worn leggings and too-small crop tops is a painful reminder of every false start. No wonder trying again feels pointless.
Fix it: But this time is different. Now she's got something she didn't have before: a plan, a purpose and you as her hype man. All she has to do is start.

12 **'I'm waiting to feel motivated.'** Waiting for the perfect moment to start is like wishing you knew tomorrow's lottery numbers. A nice thought, but it's never going to happen.
Fix it: Motivation doesn't show up until you do. If she's waiting for the stars to align, she'll be waiting for ever. But if she takes that first tiny step, she'll be amazed where the journey takes her.

Fitter and stronger together

The simple truth is that no one ever regrets getting fitter, stronger or healthier. With knowledge, confidence and encouragement – especially from you – she won't just start exercising: she'll feel more confident, more capable and more in control than she has in years.

And as you both become happier, it gets easier to reconnect, rekindle romance and put the passion back into your relationship – as you'll discover in the next chapter.

So keep showing up. Keep cheering her on. Keep reminding her why this matters so much.

Because you're not just helping her work out – you're helping her reclaim her confidence, her life, and the future you're building together.

12

Rekindle romance
Getting your love life back on track

You know how to spot the signs, have tough talks and rally medical support. You've got the tools to sleep better, stress less, move more and eat well. But there's one thing left to tackle, and it's the thing most couples never talk about.

Because when sex goes quiet, so does everything else. This chapter breaks the silence. It explains why intimacy stalls in midlife, what's really going on in both your bodies and minds, and how to bring the spark back – without pressure, shame or anxiety.

The goal isn't to get things back to how they used to be – it's to start something better.

In this chapter you'll discover:

- The main reasons sex goes missing in midlife
- Why her biggest turn-ons have changed for good
- How empathy is a direct route to enthusiasm
- Why foreplay matters more than the main event
- The eight golden rules for amazing sex for life
- How masturbation can break down intimacy barriers.

You've weathered the worst of each other's midlife mood swings, mistakes and misunderstandings. Now you're talking again. Really talking. Maybe even training together or doing things that, not long ago, felt inconceivable. Your relationship feels stronger. Like you're finally back on the same side. The reconnection is well and truly under way.

But there's still one part that feels stuck in the midlife mire. And let's be honest – you don't need us to spell it out. It's likely been on your mind for months. Or even longer.

Let's talk about sex

If only it were as simple as Salt-N-Pepa made it sound.

Most people would rather move house, get fired or swim the Channel than say those legendary lyrics out loud – unless, of course, it's 1 AM and there's a karaoke mic in hand.

But like many things in life – whether it's singing in public or admitting you're struggling – there's safety in numbers.

So let's not keep quiet any longer. Altogether now. Loud and proud: 'Let's talk about sex, baby. Let's talk about you and me.'

Why sex goes missing

Sex – by which we mean all kinds of sexual interaction, not just penetrative intercourse – is one of the most common casualties of perimenopause.[1] It's also one of the least talked about. Many women don't want to talk about it. Others don't know how. Even fewer seek help.[2] Which means their partners are often left completely in the dark – about what's happening, why it's happening, and whether it's somehow their fault.

Let's start with her. We know a lot about how women think and feel about sex, menopause and midlife thanks to the Study of Women's Health Across the Nation, or SWAN study.[3] It's one of the largest and longest-running menopause studies ever, tracking thousands of women from different ethnic and socioeconomic backgrounds since the 1990s.

Here are a few standout stats:

- Seventy-five percent of midlife women say sex is still important to them.[4]
- Nearly half of women who had no pain during sex at the start of menopause developed it within ten years of the transition beginning.[5]
- Vaginal dryness affects 19 percent of women in early perimenopause – a figure that almost doubles to 34 percent after menopause.[6]
- Most other studies agree. One meta-analysis of 54 studies, covering more than 80,000 women, found that up to 78 percent of perimenopausal women experience sexual dysfunction[7] – a term that covers a range of issues, including low desire, pain during sex, difficulty with arousal, and trouble reaching orgasm.

And, as we covered in Chapter 4, men face their own midlife challenges around sex. Around 20 percent of men in their fifties suffer from erectile dysfunction (ED)[8] – defined as struggling to get or maintain an erection – a figure that rises to almost one in two from the age of 65.[9]

ED can be caused by age-related hormone declines, but lifestyle also plays a major role. Being overweight or obese, smoking, chronic stress, poor sleep and a lack of exercise are all known factors.[10] The good news? Studies show that getting more than 150 minutes of moderate-to-vigorous exercise per week can reduce the risk of ED by up to 40 percent.[11]

From punchline to prescription

Not getting it up might be a cheap laugh in frat boy movies and old sitcoms, but it's no laughing matter in real life. It can crush confidence, chip away at self-esteem and impact your relationship. Over the long run, it's also linked to a significantly higher risk of cardiovascular disease.[12] For many men, a relatively inexpensive little blue pill can make a big difference in the moment, tackling some of the psychological and physiological barriers to sexual performance.

And this short-term solution is more popular than ever: the global ED drugs market was worth almost $3 billion (£2.2 billion) in 2024, and predicted to more than double to $7 billion by 2034.[13]

There's no quick fix for her

Women don't have the luxury of taking a pill and waiting 20 minutes for it to do the heavy lifting. The list of potential issues that can stop them thinking about, wanting or enjoying sex is far more complex, persistent, painful and often deeply distressing.

While vaginal oestrogen creams can ease some local symptoms,[14] they're only part of the picture. For many women, there are multiple barriers to overcome – physical, emotional, hormonal and psychological[15] – before the idea of sex feels anything other than upsetting, another painful reminder that she doesn't feel like the woman she used to be.

Instant expert

Dr Angela Wright on why midlife sex goes missing

Dr Angela Wright is a medical doctor and clinical sexologist who specializes in helping couples navigate sex, desire and connection through midlife and menopause. She cuts through the shame, science and social scripts to show what's really going on – and how to get the spark back.

The cultural narrative cuts deep

We're constantly surrounded by images that equate sexiness with youth. In film, TV, advertising, even pornography – it's young women who are portrayed as desirable. That narrative seeps deep into our psyches – both men and women – and reinforces the idea for many women that suddenly you're not sexy anymore.

She's not rejecting you – she's protecting herself

Sex may have become painful, or she's worried about getting a UTI. She pulls back, but not because she's gone off her partner. The message might be 'I don't want you', but that's not what she means. HRT can help, but it's not just about medication. It's about listening. About having the conversation.

Silence creates distance

Some women tell me their partner is wonderful, kind and supportive, and that they feel so guilty because he still needs something they can't give him. Others are in relationships where there's resentment – their partner's still nudging them in the night, not recognizing what's changed. The truth is, a lot of women don't talk about what's going on – they internalize it. They feel shame. Their body feels different. And then the intimacy disappears. No one's trying to reject anyone – they're trying not to hurt each other. But the silence creates distance.

Desire doesn't disappear – it evolves

Long-term monogamy, emotional burnout, resentment – for years hormones may have papered over those cracks. But when they decline, you're left facing the raw reality. If you look at the data, women in their forties report some of the most adventurous sexual fantasies. Infidelity rates rise. STIs increase in midlife. So desire doesn't disappear. It just shifts.

Think slow burn, not fast and furious

Spontaneous desire – more typical in men – is like an itch that needs scratching. Women tend to experience more responsive desire. It's not just there – it's sparked by cues: feeling safe, relaxed, seen, wanted. You put her on holiday, with some sunshine and wine, and suddenly the conditions are right. But if she's sleep-deprived, burned out, managing parents and teens, and feeling touched-out, those cues don't even register. It's like a Venn diagram: what's going on in the body, the mind, the relationship, the roles each person plays. It's different for everyone.

The 5 big barriers to sex, intimacy and connection

To move closer to the best solution, you first need to know the precise problem – because this isn't about a little bit of discomfort or simply not being in the mood. We've covered many of the most challenging perimenopause symptoms already, but here's a reminder: for many women, sex in midlife becomes a minefield of physical pain and emotional fallout. It's not just that she doesn't feel like sex – it's that her body might be actively resisting it.

Here are the five categories of symptoms that can be the reason why – and what she, you or both of you can do about it.

Direct physical symptoms

When her body's changed on the inside, it can change how sex feels or whether she wants it at all.[16]

- Thinning of the vaginal walls
- Pelvic floor weakness
- Reduced blood flow to the genitals
- Changes in clitoral sensitivity
- Loss of natural lubrication
- Tightening or shortening of the vaginal canal

What's going on?

It's oestrogen's fault, obviously. The physical effects of lower levels mean what used to feel good might now feel sore, numb, intense or completely different.

What can help?

Her body may need more time, more stimulation or more support to feel ready for sex – otherwise, what little desire she had can vanish. Water-based lube eases friction during sex, while vaginal moisturisers can be used daily to improve hydration.[17] Pelvic floor therapy can boost muscle tone and sensation,[18] and dilators can gently restore stretch and confidence after long gaps without sex.[19]

For many women, HRT is the most effective long-term option.[20] Local vaginal oestrogen (creams, pessaries or rings) can also help alongside or instead of systemic HRT.[21] Non-hormonal medications like ospemifene or vaginal DHEA may be prescribed for moderate to severe cases in the US,[22] but these types of drugs are not currently licensed for use in the UK.

Indirect physical factors

When everything else feels off – she's tired, aching or bloated – sex drops way down the list.[23]

- Joint and muscle pain
- Fatigue or chronic tiredness
- Breast tenderness
- Migraines or headaches
- Dry or itchy skin
- Bloating or digestive discomfort

What's going on?

These symptoms might not be sexual, but they're still serious mood-killers. When her body's under siege from aches, bloat, headaches or sheer exhaustion, that's all she can think about.

What can help?

It takes time. Prioritize rest, relaxation and recovery – for both of you.[24] When minds and bodies are less stressed and more fully charged, connection becomes easier.[25]

Timing matters, too. If evenings are a write-off, make space earlier in the day for joint activities that encourage low-pressure proximity – like going for a walk, training together, or even something simple like a long lunch or a trip to the pictures.

If she's constantly tired, uncomfortable and really struggling, HRT might be worth considering – if she's not on it already – to help her get back on an even keel.

Masturbation 101

The safest step back to sex?

When sex has been off the table for a while, the idea of jumping straight back into it together can feel overwhelming. So, if she's ready to get back into the swing of things, she might be better off taking matters into her own hands – at least at first.

Masturbation eased symptoms in more than a third of menopausal women, according to a Kinsey Institute study of over 1,500 women aged 40–65.[26] It improves blood flow, boosts natural lubrication, and helps rebuild that brain–body link with pleasure – especially if sex has become something she dreads rather than desires.

From flying solo to shared pleasure

As for what comes next? Mutual masturbation is linked to more positive emotions and greater sexual satisfaction for both partners, while solo-only sex, interestingly, was linked to lower satisfaction.[27] That might be because it reflects emotional distance rather than sexual connection.

Remember: hitting a home run isn't the only way to score – first, second and third base all count.

Mental and emotional reasons

If she's feeling low, lost or not like herself, sex might be the last thing on her mind.[28]

- Cognitive symptoms, like brain fog
- Chronic stress
- Irritability or mood swings
- Loss of identity
- Fear of ageing or loss of attractiveness
- Grief or sadness about fertility loss
- Performance anxiety
- Resentment or relationship friction

What's going on?
When her mood, memory, self-esteem and sense of identity are all taking a hit – and overwhelm, frustration or relationship tension are bubbling over – sex doesn't feel like an escape. It feels like another source of stress she just doesn't need.

What can help?
It's easy to take it as a personal rejection, but this is about how she feels about herself – not about you. Be patient if she's struggling with self-image or grieving the past. Focus on rebuilding trust, comfort and connection, and that starts with more honest conversations.

Therapy, coaching, journalling, or simply having more time to herself can help her reconnect with who she is now.[29] Emotional safety opens the door to physical contact. For most women in long-term relationships, emotional intimacy is the main ingredient in desire,[30] and getting it back can't be rushed.

Relationship and environmental barriers

When life is loud but your connection is quiet, intimacy runs for the hills.[31]

- Sleep deprivation
- Work or home pressure
- Checked out by caregiving
- Lack of emotional connection
- Poor communication

What's going on?

If she's exhausted, touched-out, isolated, and constantly switching between permanent parent, full-time worker, part-time carer and a dozen other roles, 'sexy night-time nymph' is a character that won't make the cut.

What can help?

Resentment kills desire faster than bad breath. No, it's not your fault if you always sleep like a baby, but doing your fair share around the house shows you're on the same wavelength. That doesn't mean you should sneak up behind her, squeeze her hips, and breathlessly whisper into her ear that you've 'just done the bins'. She might not know if you're trying to be seductive – or still catching your breath.

But pulling your weight might help more than you realize. Empathy is everything.[32] And splitting domestic duties fairly frees up space and time to do low-key things you both enjoy. It can be anything, as long as it switches off stress so other switches can turn back on.

Existential and identity shifts

If she's questioning who she is or what she wants now, sex might not make the cut.[33]

- Loss of sexual identity
- Feeling disconnected from her body
- Desire for autonomy
- Midlife reflection or regret
- Emotional disconnect
- Spiritual disconnection

What's going on?

Midlife can make us question everything – what we've done, who we are and where we're going. As we covered in Chapter 4, you're likely still working through the big questions about what comes next. So is she. Sex might feel irrelevant – or even misaligned – with who she's becoming.

What can help?

Again, don't take it personally. That's easier said than done, so focus on asking open questions – be more curious and less defensive. This is a chance to grow together, not drift apart. When she's ready, let her explore what intimacy could look like now – without pressure, judgement or assumption. Rediscovering sex as part of a new identity – not just an old habit from the past – can actually make it even more meaningful.[34]

> ### Real talk
>
> **'Humour can get you back on the same page'**
>
> *I'm Bryan. I'm 65, I'm a retired designer, and I live in Surrey.*
>
> My wife Heidi was reluctant to try HRT at first, but when a female friend developed early-onset dementia, she changed her mind and gave it a go. She started with an oestrogen gel, but she didn't get on with it. It did affect our sex life – but not in the way we hoped: she applied it before bed – so I didn't want to touch her in case I absorbed it and it shrank my bollocks!
>
> She later tried patches, but they made her nauseous, so she went back to the gel. She still applies at night, which means we now have sex in the mornings instead. I always preferred night time – especially after exercising, when my adrenaline was up – but she won that battle! She's the first to admit she's put on a bit of weight since going through the menopause but always says her breasts look great – she often jokes, 'Look at my tits, not my waist!' Nothing beats humour to break any awkwardness.

Rethinking what great sex really means

Hollywood has a lot to answer for. Forget flawless skin, perfect teeth and air-brushed bodies – its biggest crime is convincing us what great sex should look like. Add in the rise of internet porn and its endless stream of unrealistic sex, and it's no wonder so many people feel disconnected from the realities of intimacy and suffer with low sexual confidence as a result.[35]

But great sex in midlife isn't about six-packs, spontaneity or simultaneous orgasms. It's about feeling safe, wanted and close. It's about passion over performance.

Maybe it starts with holding hands or a shared bath. Maybe it doesn't even end in penetration. Maybe it's just more kissing, cuddling and closeness. That's what many midlife women say they want. Research shows that when sex becomes painful or difficult, there's often a shift in preference towards slow-burn, affection-driven intimacy – not the 'wham-bam-thank-you-Ma'am' technique you may have spent years perfecting.[36]

Every little thing you do is magic

Taking your time matters more than ever. But don't worry – this doesn't mean you should start training for all-day sex sessions that would even have Sting sweating.

Ultimately, the real foundation of a lasting sex life isn't your 'special move'. It's emotional intimacy, ongoing support and shared affection.[37]

The best first step? Ditch the pressure to pounce, perform or penetrate. If sex has started to feel like a task or a test – or has been completely missing for months – it's time to rewrite the rules. Here's your new playbook for bringing connection, comfort and curiosity – and the best sex of your life – back to the heart of your relationship.

1 **Sex isn't just penetration.** Got the message yet? We really can't stress this enough. If that's the goal every time, you're skipping over most of the menu. Prioritize connection over completion, and it might change everything.
2 **Orgasms aren't the only outcome.** We're not saying they're overrated, but for many women, they get harder to reach with age.[38] So take the pressure off her, and yourself. A great night doesn't need a grand finale. Like most things in life, the journey can be more fun than the destination.
3 **Slow beats spontaneous.** Many women don't want to be carried over your shoulder and thrown on the bed – and is that back of yours really up to it? A long, slow build-up – over days, even – makes you both feel wanted.[39] So talk: before, during and after. Tell her what you're thinking, ask what feels good, or what she'd like next time. Ditch the guesswork to build confidence and connection.

4 **Foreplay is the main event – not the warm-up.** If you treat foreplay like a box to tick, you're missing the point – and most of the pleasure. For many women, foreplay *is* sex.[40] That means slowing down, paying attention and letting things build. Words, touch, time and attention are the name of the game.
5 **Comfort comes first.** If either of you is tense, distracted or physically uncomfortable, you won't even have bad sex – let alone the mind-blowing kind. Don't soldier on when you could have set the scene. Make it comfy, calm and cosy. Lube, lighting, pillows, music, temperature and timing really do help.[41]
6 **Laugh while you're learning.** Trying something new and it not working out quite how you expected isn't failure. You don't need to examine why. This should be fun, not forensic. Laugh about it – if you can. You're rediscovering what you both like and learning what each other wants. Trial and error is part of the process.
7 **The Kama Sutra isn't a checklist.** You're not auditioning for *Cirque du Soleil*. This is about comfort and confidence, not contortionism. If you've found two or three positions that really work, use them – then explore variations from there.
8 **There's no 'normal' – only what works for you.** Forget stats, movie scripts and what social media says. The best sex in the world is the sex you're actually having – the kind that makes you feel close and desired. Whatever keeps you connected, keeps you winning.

Instant expert

Sarah Louise Ryan on how to initiate intimacy that lasts

Sarah Louise Ryan is a dating and relationship therapist who helps couples rebuild emotional and physical connection – whether they're navigating midlife transitions or looking to reignite lost sparks in a long-term relationship (sarahlouiseryan.com).

Don't sizzle when you can simmer

For many women, intimacy starts long before sex – they need time to simmer. But men often dive straight in at 11 PM, hoping for the sizzle when she's already exhausted. What she needs instead are small moments throughout the day that build connection. I call it simmering. Start by maximizing the four 'transition' moments each day that are the perfect opportunities to affirm connection and create positive relational habits. Using these moments to talk or touch creates space for closeness and builds feelings of relationship fulfilment. These important moments are:

> When you wake up: say good morning or ask how she slept.
> Before work: give her a kiss and say hope your day goes well, even if you're both at home.
> After work: ask how her day was – then really listen to what she says.
> Before bed: a kiss, a cuddle or a genuine 'I love you'.

I tell couples to try it for 30 days and watch what happens. The change is real.

Hear her love language – then speak it

Not every woman wants flowers or grand gestures. If you've been together a long time, you might think you know what she likes, but love languages can change. Don't guess. Ask. What makes her feel valued? What makes her feel seen? That's your intimacy roadmap. For some, it's quality time or kind words. For others, it's acts of service. If that's her language, then do the dishes. Change the bed. Get the groceries. If she's drowning under the domestic load, she's not going to want to rip the clothes off someone she feels she's having to parent. Do the laundry for a month and see what happens to her libido. Helping out isn't just helpful – it can be a genuine turn-on.

Change the scene to change the story

If the bedroom has become a place just for sleep – or it's associated with stress or rejection – it might not be the best place to rebuild intimacy. You may need a new environment to create new energy. A weekend away can work wonders. Even a walk somewhere unfamiliar can shift the dynamic. And when you're there, be open, honest and vulnerable. If you're feeling rejected, try saying something like, 'The story I'm telling myself is that you're not attracted to me.' It helps her understand how you feel, gives her the chance to share what's going on for her, and creates the space for a real conversation.

So what happens now?

You'll make it through the hard parts. You'll break the silence, ask the awkward questions, and start finding your way back to each other – with listening, learning and, hopefully, a lot of laughing. You rebuild your connection not by looking back – but by moving forward with a little more courage, care and clarity.

So what happens now?

Turn the page. The next chapter begins here. It's the most important one yet – but we're not the ones who get to write it.

Afterword
This isn't the end

Our chapter is over – yours is just beginning

If you've made it this far, you already know – and care – more than 99 percent of men. You understand what she's going through, how it affects every part of her life, and what you can do to help. *Really help.* And, hopefully, you've also grasped what's going on with you and started to get a clearer sense of what the second half of your life might hold and what you'd most like to be remembered for.

Right now, things might still feel out of your control. That's OK. That's normal. The menopause is a minefield – it's just that no one tells you that before you crash land here, with no warning and no map.

But keep moving. Take small steps in the right direction. You'll soon see that this isn't a no man's land after all – it's the start of something better. Together.

A changing of the seasons

In the West, the menopause is still socially and culturally tied to feelings of loss, decline and irrelevance. For many women, it feels like a slow fade into invisibility. The start of an eternal winter.

But not everywhere sees it that way.

In China, menopause is called 第二春 (*dì èr chūn*), literally translated as 'Second Spring'. It's framed as a natural and empowering transition: a new season of life, full of inner growth, wisdom and vitality.

Just across the East China Sea, Japan uses the term 更年期 (*kōnenki*) – meaning 'renewal years'. It suggests not decline, but reinvention. Not an ending, but a chance to rebalance and rediscover energy.

You're in the driving seat

With the right perspective, the menopause isn't the end of anything. It can be the start of something new: an unexpected and welcome chance to change lanes, right at the moment you both thought you'd run out of road.

So keep your foot on the gas. Keep talking. Keep showing up.

Because the everyday hero she needs?

He's already here.

References

Chapter 1

1. https://www.benenden.co.uk/newsroom/quarter-of-men-dont-know-what-the-menopause-is/
2. British Menopause Society (2023). *What is the menopause?* https://thebms.org.uk/wp-content/uploads/2023/08/17-BMS-TfC-What-is-the-menopause-AUGUST2023-A.pdf
3. www.wellbeingofwomen.org.uk/news/new-data-reveals-big-gap-in-access-to-hormone-replacement-therapy-for-ethnic-minority-and-deprived-women/
4. https://www.letstalkmenopause.org/
5. Panay, N., Ang, S. B., Cheshire, R., Goldstein, S. R., Maki, P., Nappi, R. E. and International Menopause Society Board (2024). Menopause and MHT in 2024: addressing the key controversies: an International Menopause Society White Paper. *South African General Practitioner*, 5(3), 119–34.
6. https://www.independent.co.uk/news/uk/home-news/perimenopause-suicidal-thoughts-menopause-mental-health-b1933346.html
7. Brinton, R. D., Yao, J., Yin, F., Mack, W. J. and Cadenas, E. (2015). Perimenopause as a neurological transition state. *Nature Reviews Endocrinology*, 11(7), 393–405.
8. https://www.nhs.uk/conditions/menopause/symptoms
9. National Institute for Health and Care Excellence (NICE) (2015). *Menopause: Diagnosis and management (NICE Guideline NG23)*. https://www.nice.org.uk/guidance/ng23
10. Mishra, G. D., Davies, M. C., Hillman, S., Chung, H. F., Roy, S., Maclaran, K. and Hickey, M. (2024). Optimising health after early menopause. *The Lancet*, 403(10430), 958–68.
11. Barber, K. and Charles, A. (2023). Barriers to accessing effective treatment and support for menopausal symptoms: a qualitative study capturing the behaviours, beliefs and experiences of key stakeholders. *Patient Preference and Adherence*, 2971–80.
12. Harper, J., Keay, N., Rowe, F., Alstyne, P. V. and Tariq, S. (2024). The time has come for a UK-wide menopause education and support programme: InTune. *Women's Health*, 20, 17455057241277535.
13. https://menopausesupport.co.uk/?p=3870#
14. Keay, N. (2024). *Myths of Menopause: A guide to increasing your menopause wisdom*. Sequoia Hammersmith Books.
15. Tariq, B., Phillips, S., Biswakarma, R., Talaulikar, V. and Harper, J. C. (2023). Women's knowledge and attitudes to the menopause:

a comparison of women over 40 who were in the perimenopause, post menopause and those not in the peri or post menopause. *BMC Women's Health, 23*(1), 460.
16 Ibid.
17 Parish, S. J., Faubion, S. S., Weinberg, M., Bernick, B. and Mirkin, S. (2019). The MATE survey: men's perceptions and attitudes towards menopause and their role in partners' menopausal transition. *Menopause, 26*(10), 1110–16.
18 https://www.stowefamilylaw.co.uk/stowe-support/menopause-a-divorce-danger-zone/
19 https://www.balance-menopause.com/news/menopause-puts-final-nail-in-marriage-coffin
20 https://www.aarp.org/pri/topics/social-leisure/relationships/divorce/
21 Danzebrink, D. (2018). *Making Menopause Matter: The essential guide to what you need to know and why.* Sheldon Press.
22 Abernethy, K. (2017). *Menopause: The one-stop guide.* Souvenir Press.

Chapter 2

1 Nussey, S. and Whitehead, S. (2001). Principles of endocrinology. *Endocrinology: An integrated approach, 1–21*; https://www.endocrine.org/patient-engagement/endocrine-library/hormones-and-endocrine-function
2 Sharpe, R. M. (1998). The roles of oestrogen in the male. *Trends in Endocrinology & Metabolism, 9*(9), 371–7.
3 Reed, B. G. and Carr, B. R. (2015). The normal menstrual cycle and the control of ovulation. *Endotext* [Internet]. South Dartmouth.
4 Thau, L., Gandhi, J. and Sharma, S. (2023). Physiology, cortisol. In *StatPearls* [Internet]. StatPearls Publishing.
5 Aulinas, A. (2019). Physiology of the pineal gland and melatonin. *Endotext* [Internet]. South Dartmouth.
6 Rahman, M. S., Hossain, K. S., Das, S., Kundu, S., Adegoke, E. O., Rahman, M. A., ... and Pang, M. G. (2021). Role of insulin in health and disease: an update. *International Journal of Molecular Sciences, 22*(12), 6403.
7 Hall, J. E. (2015). Endocrinology of the menopause. *Endocrinology and Metabolism Clinics, 44*(3), 485–96.
8 Woods, N. F., Mitchell, E. S. and Smith-DiJulio, K. (2009). Cortisol levels during the menopausal transition and early postmenopause: observations from the Seattle Midlife Women's Health Study. *Menopause, 16*(4), 708–18.
9 Jehan, S., Jean-Louis, G., Zizi, F., Auguste, E., Pandi-Perumal, S. R., Gupta, R., ... and Brzezinski, A. (2017). Sleep, melatonin, and the menopausal transition: what are the links? *Sleep Science, 10*(01), 11–18.

10 Genazzani, A. D., Petrillo, T., Semprini, E., Aio, C., Foschi, M., Ambrosetti, F., ... and Battipaglia, C. (2024). Metabolic syndrome, insulin resistance and menopause: the changes in body structure and the therapeutic approach. *Gynecological and Reproductive Endocrinology & Metabolism, 4*, 86–91.
11 Davis, S. R., Pinkerton, J., Santoro, N. and Simoncini, T. (2023). Menopause: biology, consequences, supportive care, and therapeutic options. *Cell, 186*(19), 4038–58.
12 Ibid.
13 https://www.nice.org.uk/guidance/ng23
14 Cable, J. K. and Grider, M. H. (2023). Physiology, progesterone. [Updated 2023 May 1.] *StatPearls* [Internet]. StatPearls Publishing.
15 Nassar, G. N. and Leslie, S. W. (2018). Physiology, testosterone. https://www.ncbi.nlm.nih.gov/books/NBK526128/
16 Panay, N. and British Menopause Society (2022). *Testosterone replacement in menopause: Tool for clinicians – Information for GPs and other health professionals.* British Menopause Society. https://www.womens-health-concern.org/help-and-advice/factsheets/testosterone-for-women/
17 Del Río, J. P., Alliende, M. I., Molina, N., Serrano, F. G., Molina, S. and Vigil, P. (2018). Steroid hormones and their action in women's brains: the importance of hormonal balance. *Frontiers in Public Health, 6*, 141.
18 Handelsman, D. J., Sikaris, K. and Ly, L. P. (2016). Estimating age-specific trends in circulating testosterone and sex hormone-binding globulin in males and females across the lifespan. *Annals of Clinical Biochemistry, 53*(3), 377–84.
19 https://womenshealth.gov/menstrual-cycle/premenstrual-syndrome; https://www.nhs.uk/conditions/pre-menstrual-syndrome/
20 https://www.nhs.uk/conditions/menopause/symptoms/
21 Santoro, N., Roeca, C., Peters, B. A. and Neal-Perry, G. (2021). The menopause transition: signs, symptoms, and management options. *The Journal of Clinical Endocrinology & Metabolism, 106*(1), 1–15.
22 https://www.nhs.uk/conditions/menopause/
23 https://www.engage.england.nhs.uk/safety-and-innovation/menopause-in-the-workplace
24 https://womenshealth.gov/menopause/early-or-premature-menopause
25 Santoro, N., Roeca, C., Peters, B. A. and Neal-Perry, G. (2021). The menopause transition: signs, symptoms, and management options. *The Journal of Clinical Endocrinology & Metabolism, 106*(1), 1–15.
26 Koothirezhi, R. and Ranganathan, S. (2020). Postmenopausal syndrome. https://www.ncbi.nlm.nih.gov/books/NBK560840/
27 https://www.nhs.uk/conditions/early-or-premature-menopause/

28 https://womenshealth.gov/menopause/early-or-premature-menopause
29 https://www.nhs.uk/conditions/early-or-premature-menopause/
30 Okeke, T. C., Anyaehie, U. B. and Ezenyeaku, C. C. (2013). Premature menopause. *Annals of Medical and Health Sciences Research*, *3*(1), 90–5.
31 British Menopause Society (2024). *Talking about surgical menopause.* https://thebms.org.uk/wp-content/uploads/2024/10/13-BMS-TfC-Surgical-Menopause-SEPT2024-D.pdf
32 Davis, S. R., Pinkerton, J., Santoro, N. and Simoncini, T. (2023). Menopause: biology, consequences, supportive care, and therapeutic options. *Cell*, *186*(19), 4038–58.
33 Chen, P., Li, B. and Ou-Yang, L. (2022). Role of estrogen receptors in health and disease. *Frontiers in Endocrinology*, *13*, 839005.
34 Ibid.
35 https://www.nhs.uk/conditions/menopause/symptoms/; Burbos, N. and Morris, E. P. (2011). Menopausal symptoms. *BMJ Clinical Evidence*, 0804; Santoro, N. (2016). Perimenopause: from research to practice. *Journal of Women's Health*, *25*(4), 332–9; Mishra, G. D. and Kuh, D. (2012). Health symptoms during midlife in relation to menopausal transition: British prospective cohort study. *British Medical Journal*, *344*.
36 Brinton, R. D., Yao, J., Yin, F., Mack, W. J. and Cadenas, E. (2015). Perimenopause as a neurological transition state. *Nature Reviews Endocrinology*, *11*(7), 393–405.
37 https://www.independent.co.uk/news/uk/home-news/perimenopause-suicidal-thoughts-menopause-mental-health-b1933346.html
38 Fawcett Society (2022). Menopause in the workplace: impact on women in the UK. https://www.fawcettsociety.org.uk/Handlers/Download.ashx?IDMF=9672cf45-5f13-4b69-8882-1e5e643ac8a6
39 Bansal, R. and Aggarwal, N. (2019). Menopausal hot flashes: a concise review. *Journal of Mid-Life Health*, *10*(1), 6–13; Morrow, P. K. H., Mattair, D. N. and Hortobagyi, G. N. (2011). Hot flashes: a review of pathophysiology and treatment modalities. *The Oncologist*, *16*(11), 1658–64.
40 https://www.bupa.co.uk/newsroom/ourviews/symptoms-menopause-hot-flushes
41 Zhang, Z., DiVittorio, J. R., Joseph, A. M. and Correa, S. M. (2021). The effects of estrogens on neural circuits that control temperature. *Endocrinology*, *162*(8), bqab087.
42 https://www.nia.nih.gov/health/menopause/hot-flashes-what-can-i-do
43 Thurston, R. C. and Joffe, H. (2011). Vasomotor symptoms and menopause: findings from the Study of Women's Health across the Nation. *Obstetrics and Gynecology Clinics of North America*, *38*(3), 489.

44 Cameron, C. R., Cohen, S., Sewell, K. and Lee, M. (2024). The art of hormone replacement therapy (HRT) in menopause management. *Journal of Pharmacy Practice, 37*(3), 736–40.

45 https://thebms.org.uk/2023/12/new-treatment-for-vasomotor-symptoms-hot-flushes-and-night-sweats-licensed-by-the-mhra/; https://www.nhs.uk/medicines/hormone-replacement-therapy-hrt/alternatives-to-hormone-replacement-therapy-hrt/other-medicines-for-menopause-symptoms/

46 Norton, S., Chilcot, J. and Hunter, M. S. (2014). Cognitive-behavior therapy for menopausal symptoms (hot flushes and night sweats): moderators and mediators of treatment effects. *Menopause, 21*(6), 574–8; Mann, E., Smith, M. J., Hellier, J., Balabanovic, J. A., Hamed, H., Grunfeld, E. A. and Hunter, M. S. (2012). Cognitive behavioural treatment for women who have menopausal symptoms after breast cancer treatment (MENOS 1): a randomised controlled trial. *The Lancet Oncology, 13*(3), 309–18.

47 Fawcett Society (2022). Menopause in the workplace: impact on women in the UK. https://www.fawcettsociety.org.uk/Handlers/Download.ashx?IDMF=9672cf45-5f13-4b69-8882-1e5e643ac8a6

48 Greendale, G. A., Huang, M. H., Wight, R. G., Seeman, T., Luetters, C., Avis, N. E., ... and Karlamangla, A. S. (2009). Effects of the menopause transition and hormone use on cognitive performance in midlife women. *Neurology, 72*(21), 1850–7.

49 Ramadhana, D. R., Putra, R. P., Sibarani, M. A., Sulistiawati, S., Sari, D. R., Rejeki, P. S., ... and Argarini, R. (2024). Short-term multicomponent exercise training improves executive function in postmenopausal women. *PLOS One, 19*(8), e0307812; Gava, G., Orsili, I., Alvisi, S., Mancini, I., Seracchioli, R. and Meriggiola, M. C. (2019). Cognition, mood and sleep in menopausal transition: the role of menopause hormone therapy. *Medicina, 55*(10), 668.

50 Girard, R., Météreau, E., Thomas, J., Pugeat, M., Qu, C. and Dreher, J. C. (2017). Hormone therapy at early post-menopause increases cognitive control-related prefrontal activity. *Scientific Reports, 7*(1), 44917.

51 Fawcett Society (2022). Menopause in the workplace: impact on women in the UK. https://www.fawcettsociety.org.uk/Handlers/Download.ashx?IDMF=9672cf45-5f13-4b69-8882-1e5e643ac8a6

52 https://www.mind.org.uk/information-support/tips-for-everyday-living/menopause-and-mental-health/how-can-menopause-affect-mental-health/#FeelingAnxious

53 Stute, P. and Lozza-Fiacco, S. (2022). Strategies to cope with stress and anxiety during the menopausal transition. *Maturitas, 166*, 1–13; Kandasamy, G., Almaghaslah, D. and Almanasef, M. (2024). A study on

anxiety and depression symptoms among menopausal women: a web based cross sectional survey. *Frontiers in Public Health, 12*, 1467731.
54 Stute, P. and Lozza-Fiacco, S. (2022). Strategies to cope with stress and anxiety during the menopausal transition. *Maturitas, 166*, 1–13.
55 Fawcett Society (2022). Menopause in the workplace: impact on women in the UK. https://www.fawcettsociety.org.uk/Handlers/Download.ashx?IDMF=9672cf45-5f13-4b69-8882-1e5e643ac8a6
56 Troìa, L., Garassino, M., Volpicelli, A. I., Fornara, A., Libretti, A., Surico, D. and Remorgida, V. (2025). Sleep disturbance and perimenopause: a narrative review. *Journal of Clinical Medicine, 14*(5), 1479.
57 Zeng, W., Xu, J., Yang, Y., Lv, M. and Chu, X. (2025). Factors influencing sleep disorders in perimenopausal women: a systematic review and meta-analysis. *Frontiers in Neurology, 16*, 1460613.
58 Ibid.
59 Drake, C. L., Kalmbach, D. A., Arnedt, J. T., Cheng, P., Tonnu, C. V., Cuamatzi-Castelan, A. and Fellman-Couture, C. (2019). Treating chronic insomnia in postmenopausal women: a randomized clinical trial comparing cognitive-behavioral therapy for insomnia, sleep restriction therapy, and sleep hygiene education. *Sleep, 42*(2), zsy217.
60 Rusch, H. L., Rosario, M., Levison, L. M., Olivera, A., Livingston, W. S., Wu, T. and Gill, J. M. (2019). The effect of mindfulness meditation on sleep quality: a systematic review and meta-analysis of randomized controlled trials. *Annals of the New York Academy of Sciences, 1445*(1), 5–16; Sucu, C. and Çitil, E. T. (2024). The effect of progressive muscle relaxation exercises on postmenopausal sleep quality and fatigue: a single-blind randomized controlled study. *Menopause, 31*(8), 669–78.
61 Qian, J., Sun, S., Wang, M., Sun, Y., Sun, X., Jevitt, C. and Yu, X. (2023). The effect of exercise intervention on improving sleep in menopausal women: a systematic review and meta-analysis. *Frontiers in Medicine, 10*, 1092294; Kline, C. E., Irish, L. A., Krafty, R. T., Sternfeld, B., Kravitz, H. M., Buysse, D. J., ... and Hall, M. H. (2013). Consistently high sports/exercise activity is associated with better sleep quality, continuity and depth in midlife women: the SWAN sleep study. *Sleep, 36*(9), 1279–88.
62 McCurry, S. M., Guthrie, K. A., Morin, C. M., Woods, N. F., Landis, C. A., Ensrud, K. E., ... and LaCroix, A. Z. (2016). Telephone-based cognitive behavioral therapy for insomnia in perimenopausal and postmenopausal women with vasomotor symptoms: a MsFLASH randomized clinical trial. *JAMA Internal Medicine, 176*(7), 913–20.
63 Silva, B. H., Martinez, D. and Wender, M. C. O. (2011). A randomized, controlled pilot trial of hormone therapy for menopausal insomnia. *Archives of Women's Mental Health, 14*, 505–8.

64 Fawcett Society (2022). Menopause in the workplace: impact on women in the UK. https://www.fawcettsociety.org.uk/Handlers/Download.ashx?IDMF=9672cf45-5f13-4b69-8882-1e5e643ac8a6

65 Carlson, K. and Nguyen, H. (2024). Genitourinary syndrome of menopause. In *StatPearls* [Internet]. StatPearls Publishing.

66 Basson, R. (2010). Testosterone therapy for reduced libido in women. *Therapeutic Advances in Endocrinology and Metabolism*, *1*(4), 155–64.

67 Edwards, D. and Panay, N. (2016). Treating vulvovaginal atrophy/genitourinary syndrome of menopause: how important is vaginal lubricant and moisturizer composition? *Climacteric*, *19*(2), 151–61.

68 Falgares, G., Costanzo, G., Fontanesi, L., Verrocchio, M. C., Bin, F. and Marchetti, D. (2024). The role of sexual communication in the relationship between emotion regulation and sexual functioning in women: the impact of age and relationship status. *International Journal of Clinical and Health Psychology*, *24*(3), 100482.

69 Cameron, C. R., Cohen, S., Sewell, K. and Lee, M. (2024). The art of hormone replacement therapy (HRT) in menopause management. *Journal of Pharmacy Practice*, *37*(3), 736–40.

70 https://www.nhs.uk/medicines/hormone-replacement-therapy-hrt/vaginal-oestrogen/about-vaginal-oestrogen/

71 https://www.nhs.uk/conditions/menopause/treatment/

Chapter 3

1 Newson, L. (2023). *The Definitive Guide to the Perimenopause and Menopause*. Yellow Kite; Newson, L. (2021). *Preparing for the Perimenopause and Menopause*. Penguin Life.

2 Muir, K. (2022). *Everything You Need to Know about the Menopause (But Were Too Afraid to Ask)*. Gallery UK.

3 https://www.endocrine.org/patient-engagement/endocrine-library/hormones-and-endocrine-function/reproductive-hormones

4 Tariq, B., Phillips, S., Biswakarma, R., Talaulikar, V. and Harper, J. C. (2023). Women's knowledge and attitudes to the menopause: a comparison of women over 40 who were in the perimenopause, post menopause and those not in the peri or post menopause. *BMC Women's Health*, *23*(1), 460.

5 Nosek, M., Kennedy, H. P. and Gudmundsdottir, M. (2010). Silence, stigma, and shame: a postmodern analysis of distress during menopause. *Advances in Nursing Science*, *33*(3), E24–E36.

6 Simmons, K., Llewellyn, C., Bremner, S., Gilleece, Y., Norcross, C. and Iwuji, C. (2024). The barriers and enablers to accessing sexual health and sexual well-being services for midlife women (aged 40–65 years) in

high-income countries: a mixed-methods systematic review. *Women's Health*, 20, 17455057241277723.
7   Moon, D. U., Kim, H., Jung, J. H., Han, K. and Jeon, H. J. (2024). Association of age at menopause and suicide risk in postmenopausal women: a nationwide cohort study. *Frontiers in Psychiatry*, 15, 1442991.
8   https://www.ons.gov.uk/peoplepopulationandcommunity/birthsdeathsandmarriages/deaths/bulletins/suicidesintheunitedkingdom/2023
9   https://www.balance-menopause.com/news/menopause-puts-final-nail-in-marriage-coffin/
10 Aras, S. G., Grant, A. D. and Konhilas, J. P. (2025). Clustering of >145,000 symptom logs reveals distinct pre, peri, and menopausal phenotypes. *Scientific Reports*, 15(1), 640.
11 Wang, X., Wang, L., Di, J., Zhang, X. and Zhao, G. (2021). Prevalence and risk factors for menopausal symptoms in middle-aged Chinese women: a community-based cross-sectional study. *Menopause*, 28(11), 1271–8.
12 Rowe-Ham, K. (2023). *Owning Your Menopause: Fitter, calmer, stronger in 30 days*. Yellow Kite.
13 Zhang, Z., DiVittorio, J. R., Joseph, A. M. and Correa, S. M. (2021). The effects of estrogens on neural circuits that control temperature. *Endocrinology*, 162(8), bqab087.
14 Bendis, P. C., Zimmerman, S., Onisiforou, A., Zanos, P. and Georgiou, P. (2024). The impact of estradiol on serotonin, glutamate, and dopamine systems. *Frontiers in Neuroscience*, 18, 1348551.
15 Russell, J. K., Jones, C. K. and Newhouse, P. A. (2019). The role of estrogen in brain and cognitive aging. *Neurotherapeutics*, 16(3), 649–65.
16 Brinton, R. D., Yao, J., Yin, F., Mack, W. J. and Cadenas, E. (2015). Perimenopause as a neurological transition state. *Nature Reviews Endocrinology*, 11(7), 393–405.
17 Meziou, N., Scholfield, C., Taylor, C. A. and Armstrong, H. L. (2023). Hormone therapy for sexual function in perimenopausal and postmenopausal women: a systematic review and meta-analysis update. *Menopause*, 30(6), 659–71.
18 Astrup, K., Olivarius, N. D. F., Møller, S., Gottschau, A. and Karlslund, W. (2004). Menstrual bleeding patterns in pre- and perimenopausal women: a population-based prospective diary study. *Acta Obstetricia et Gynecologica Scandinavica*, 83(2), 197–202.
19 Bendis, P. C., Zimmerman, S., Onisiforou, A., Zanos, P. and Georgiou, P. (2024). The impact of estradiol on serotonin, glutamate, and dopamine systems. *Frontiers in Neuroscience*, 18, 1348551.
20 https://www.health.harvard.edu/womens-health/why-has-my-natural-scent-changed-during-perimenopause

21 https://www.mumsnet.com/talk/menopause/3129245-Perimenopause-and-Sex-Surge

Chapter 4

1. https://www.nhs.uk/conditions/male-menopause/
2. Kraemer, W. J. and Ratamess, N. A. (2005). Hormonal responses and adaptations to resistance exercise and training. *Sports Medicine, 35*, 339–61.
3. Martinez Kercher, V. M., Watkins, J. M., Goss, J. M., Phillips, L. A., Roy, B. A., Blades, K., ... and Kercher, K. A. (2024). Psychological needs, self-efficacy, motivation, and resistance training outcomes in a 16-week barbell training program for adults. *Frontiers in Psychology, 15*, 1439431.
4. Neumann, R. J., Ahrens, K. F., Kollmann, B., Goldbach, N., Chmitorz, A., Weichert, D., ... and Matura, S. (2022). The impact of physical fitness on resilience to modern life stress and the mediating role of general self-efficacy. *European Archives of Psychiatry and Clinical Neuroscience*, 1–14.
5. https://www.endocrine.org/patient-engagement/endocrine-library/hormones-and-endocrine-function/reproductive-hormones
6. Straftis, A. A. and Gray, P. B. (2019). Sex, energy, well-being and low testosterone: an exploratory survey of US men's experiences on prescription testosterone. *International Journal of Environmental Research and Public Health, 16*(18), 3261.
7. https://www.endocrine.org/patient-engagement/endocrine-library/hormones-and-endocrine-function/reproductive-hormones
8. Yang, Q., Li, Z., Li, W., Lu, L., Wu, H., Zhuang, Y., ... and Sui, X. (2019). Association of total testosterone, free testosterone, bioavailable testosterone, sex hormone-binding globulin, and hypertension. *Medicine, 98*(20), e15628.
9. Straftis, A. A. and Gray, P. B. (2019). Sex, energy, well-being and low testosterone: an exploratory survey of US men's experiences on prescription testosterone. *International Journal of Environmental Research and Public Health, 16*(18), 3261.
10. https://www.endocrine.org/patient-engagement/endocrine-library/hypogonadism
11. Traish, A. M., Miner, M. M., Morgentaler, A. and Zitzmann, M. (2011). Testosterone deficiency. *The American Journal of Medicine, 124*(7), 578–87.
12. https://www.endocrine.org/patient-engagement/endocrine-library/hypogonadism
13. Morales, A., Bebb, R. A., Manjoo, P., Assimakopoulos, P., Axler, J., Collier, C., ... and Lee, J. C. (2015). Diagnosis and management of testosterone deficiency syndrome in men: clinical practice guideline. *Cmaj, 187*(18), 1369–77.

14 Mulligan, T., Frick, M. F., Zuraw, Q. C., Stemhagen, A. and McWhirter, C. (2006). Prevalence of hypogonadism in males aged at least 45 years: the HIM study. *International Journal of Clinical Practice*, 60(7), 762–9.
15 https://www.health.harvard.edu/mens-health/lifestyle-strategies-to-help-prevent-natural-age-related-decline-in-testosterone
16 Cho, D. Y., Yeo, J. K., Cho, S. I., Jung, J. E., Yang, S. J., Kong, D. H., ... and Park, M. G. (2017). Exercise improves the effects of testosterone replacement therapy and the durability of response after cessation of treatment: a pilot randomized controlled trial. *Asian Journal of Andrology*, 19(5), 602–7.
17 Straftis, A. A. and Gray, P. B. (2019). Sex, energy, well-being and low testosterone: an exploratory survey of US men's experiences on prescription testosterone. *International Journal of Environmental Research and Public Health*, 16(18), 3261.
18 Straftis, A. A. and Gray, P. B. (2019). Sex, energy, well-being and low testosterone: an exploratory survey of US men's experiences on prescription testosterone. *International Journal of Environmental Research and Public Health*, 16(18), 3261.
19 https://www.manual.co/blog/testosterone-replacement-therapy-trt-in-the-uk
20 Chu, B., Marwaha, K., Sanvictores, T., Awosika, A. O. and Ayers, D. (2024). Physiology, stress reaction. In *StatPearls* [Internet]. StatPearls Publishing.
21 Lim, S. Y., Ha, H. S., Kwon, H. S., Lee, J. H., Yim, H. W., Yoon, K. H., ... and Park, Y. M. (2011). Factors associated with insulin resistance in a middle-aged non-obese rural population: the Chungju Metabolic Disease Cohort (CMC) Study. *Epidemiology and Health*, 33, e2011009; Singh, M. (2014). Mood, food, and obesity. *Frontiers in Psychology*, 5, 925.
22 Rod, T., Nieschlag, E., Kanakis, G., Maggi, M., Gooren, L., Dean, J. D., Giwercman, A., Kicovic, P., Ramasamy, R., Saad, F. and Wu, F. C. W. (2023). EMAS position statement: testosterone replacement therapy in older men. *Maturitas*, 175, 107781; https://www.maturitas.org/action/showPdf?pii=S0378-5122%2823%2900460-7
23 Hackett, G., Kirby, M., Rees, R. W., Jones, T. H., Muneer, A., Livingston, M., ... and Ramachandran, S. (2023). The British Society for Sexual Medicine guidelines on male adult testosterone deficiency, with statements for practice. *The World Journal of Men's Health*, 41(3), 508.
24 Petering, R. C. and Brooks, N. A. (2017). Testosterone therapy: review of clinical applications. *American Family Physician*, 96(7), 441–9.
25 Bassil, N., Alkaade, S. and Morley, J. E. (2009). The benefits and risks of testosterone replacement therapy: a review. *Therapeutics and Clinical Risk Management*, 427–48.

26 Jasuja, G. K., Bhasin, S., Rose, A. J., Reisman, J. I., Hanlon, J. T., Miller, D. R., ... and Berlowitz, D. R. (2017). Provider and site-level determinants of testosterone prescribing in the veterans healthcare system. *The Journal of Clinical Endocrinology & Metabolism, 102*(9), 3226–33.
27 Leproult, R. and Van Cauter, E. (2011). Effect of 1 week of sleep restriction on testosterone levels in young healthy men. *Jama, 305*(21), 2173–4.
28 Hirokawa, K., Fujii, Y., Taniguchi, T. and Tsujishita, M. (2022). Associations of testosterone and cortisol concentrations with sleep quality in Japanese male workers. *Comprehensive Psychoneuroendocrinology, 12*, 100158.
29 Okobi, O. E., Khoury, P., Raul, J., Figueroa, R. S., Desai, D., Mangiliman, B. D. A., ... and Borges, S. H. (2024). Impact of weight loss on testosterone levels: a review of BMI and testosterone. *Cureus, 16*(12).
30 Anders, S. M. van (2012). Testosterone and sexual desire in healthy women and men. *Archives of Sexual Behavior, 41*, 1471–84.
31 https://www.health.harvard.edu/mens-health/lifestyle-strategies-to-help-prevent-natural-age-related-decline-in-testosterone
32 Mües, H. M., Markert, C., Feneberg, A. C. and Nater, U. M. (2025). Bidirectional associations between daily subjective stress and sexual desire, arousal, and activity in healthy men and women. *Annals of Behavioral Medicine, 59*(1), kaaf007.
33 Thornton, K., Chervenak, J. and Neal-Perry, G. (2015). Menopause and sexuality. *Endocrinology and Metabolism Clinics, 44*(3), 649–61.
34 Thomas, H. M., Bryce, C. L., Ness, R. B. and Hess, R. (2011). Dyspareunia is associated with decreased frequency of intercourse in the menopausal transition. *Menopause, 18*(2), 152–7.
35 https://www.medicalnewstoday.com/articles/sex-drive#summary
36 Adebisi, O. Y. and Carlson, K. (2024). *Female Sexual Interest and Arousal Disorder*. StatPearls Publishing.
37 Infurna, F. J., Gerstorf, D. and Lachman, M. E. (2020). Midlife in the 2020s: opportunities and challenges. *American Psychologist, 75*(4), 470.
38 Eriksen, C. B. (2021). Men in/and crisis: the cultural narrative of men's midlife crises. *Journal of Aging Studies, 57*, 100926.
39 Brooks, D. (2019). *The Second Mountain: The quest for a moral life*. Allen Lane (UK) / Random House (US).
40 Biglan, A., Van Ryzin, M. J., Moore, K. J., Mauricci, M. and Mannan, I. (2019). The socialization of boys and men in the modern era: an evolutionary mismatch. *Development and Psychopathology, 31*(5), 1789–99.
41 Hackett, G., Kirby, M., Edwards, D., Jones, T. H., Wylie, K., Ossei-Gerning, N., ... and Muneer, A. (2017). British Society for Sexual Medicine guidelines on adult testosterone deficiency, with statements for UK practice. *The Journal of Sexual Medicine, 14*(12), 1504–23.

42 https://www.auanet.org/guidelines-and-quality/guidelines/testosterone-deficiency-guideline
43 American Urological Association (2023). Evaluation and management of testosterone deficiency: AUA guideline. https://www.auanet.org/documents/Guidelines/PDF/Testosterone percent20Website percent20Final percent280 percent29.pdf
44 https://www.imarcgroup.com/testosterone-replacement-therapy-market
45 Straftis, A. A. and Gray, P. B. (2019). Sex, energy, well-being and low testosterone: an exploratory survey of US men's experiences on prescription testosterone. *International Journal of Environmental Research and Public Health*, 16(18), 3261.
46 Farber, N. J., Vij, S. C. and Shoskes, D. A. (2020). Failure of testosterone replacement therapy to improve symptoms correlates with burden of systemic conditions. *Translational Andrology and Urology*, 9(3), 1108.
47 https://www.ncic.nhs.uk/patients-visitors/patient-information-leaflets/Testosterone-replacement-therapy
48 Liu, V. N., Johnson, H., Huang, D., Clift, A. K., Alaa, A. and El-Osta, A. (2025). A qualitative exploration of testosterone replacement therapy: men's experiences and healthcare barriers. *Trends in Urology & Men's Health*, 16(3), e12007.
49 Jung, C. G. (1959). *The Archetypes and the Collective Unconscious.* Princeton University Press.
50 Lars Tornstam (2005). *Gerotranscendence: A developmental theory of positive aging.* Springer.
51 Hackett, G., Kirby, M., Edwards, D., Jones, T. H., Rees, J. and Muneer, A. (2017). UK policy statements on testosterone deficiency. *International Journal of Clinical Practice*, 71(3–4), e12901.
52 Saad, Farid, et al. (2011). Onset of effects of testosterone treatment and time span until maximum effects are achieved. *European Journal of Endocrinology*, 165(5), 675–85.
53 https://www.ncic.nhs.uk/patients-visitors/patient-information-leaflets/Testosterone-replacement-therapy
54 https://www.manual.co/blog/testosterone-replacement-therapy-trt-in-the-uk
55 https://honehealth.com/edge/testosterone-replacement-therapy-cost/
56 Petering, R. C. and Brooks, N. A. (2017). Testosterone therapy: review of clinical applications. *American Family Physician*, 96(7), 441–9.
57 Osterberg, E. C., Bernie, A. M. and Ramasamy, R. (2014). Risks of testosterone replacement therapy in men. *Indian Journal of Urology*, 30(1), 2–7.
58 Ibid.

59 Suetomi, T., Ichioka, D., Iimura, T., Kojo, K., Ikeda, A., Kimura, T., ... and Nishiyama, H. (2022). Characteristics of testicular atrophy during testosterone replacement therapy (TRT). *The Journal of Sexual Medicine*, *19*(5), S175.
60 https://themenshealthclinic.co.uk/trt-best-practice/
61 Millar, A. C., Lau, A. N., Tomlinson, G., Kraguljac, A., Simel, D. L., Detsky, A. S. and Lipscombe, L. L. (2016). Predicting low testosterone in aging men: a systematic review. *Cmaj*, *188*(13), E321–E330.
62 Hackett, G., Kirby, M., Edwards, D., Jones, T. H., Wylie, K., Ossei-Gerning, N., ... and Muneer, A. (2017). British Society for Sexual Medicine guidelines on adult testosterone deficiency, with statements for UK practice. *The Journal of Sexual Medicine*, *14*(12), 1504–23.
63 https://www.apa.org/monitor/2023/11/navigating-late-in-life-divorce

Chapter 5

1 Cavendish, L. (2023). *How to Have Extraordinary Relationships*. Piatkus.
2 Kozlowska, K., Walker, P., McLean, L. and Carrive, P. (2015). Fear and the defense cascade: clinical implications and management. *Harvard Review of Psychiatry*, *23*(4), 263–87.
3 Chu, B., Marwaha, K., Sanvictores, T., Awosika, A. O. and Ayers, D. (2024). Physiology, stress reaction. In *StatPearls* [Internet]. StatPearls Publishing.
4 Meier, J. K. and Schwabe, L. (2024). Consistently increased dorsolateral prefrontal cortex activity during the exposure to acute stressors. *Cerebral Cortex*, *34*(4), bhae159.
5 Thayer, J. F. and Lane, R. D. (2000). A model of neurovisceral integration in emotion regulation and dysregulation. *Journal of Affective Disorders*, *61*(3), 201–16.
6 Ma, X., Yue, Z. Q., Gong, Z. Q., Zhang, H., Duan, N. Y., Shi, Y. T., ... and Li, Y. F. (2017). The effect of diaphragmatic breathing on attention, negative affect and stress in healthy adults. *Frontiers in Psychology*, *8*, 234806.
7 McEwen, B. S. (2007). Physiology and neurobiology of stress and adaptation: central role of the brain. *Physiological Reviews*, *87*(3), 873–904; Yoo, S. S., Gujar, N., Hu, P., Jolesz, F. A. and Walker, M. P. (2007). The human emotional brain without sleep: a prefrontal amygdala disconnect. *Current Biology*, *17*(20), R877–R878.
8 Arnsten, A. F. (2009). Stress signalling pathways that impair prefrontal cortex structure and function. *Nature Reviews Neuroscience*, *10*(6), 410–22.
9 Balban, M. Y., Neri, E., Kogon, M. M., Weed, L., Nouriani, B., Jo, B., ... and Huberman, A. D. (2023). Brief structured respiration practices enhance mood and reduce physiological arousal. *Cell Reports Medicine*, *4*(1).
10 Zaccaro, A., Piarulli, A., Laurino, M., Garbella, E., Menicucci, D., Neri, B. and Gemignani, A. (2018). How breath-control can change your

life: a systematic review on psycho-physiological correlates of slow breathing. *Frontiers in Human Neuroscience, 12*, 409421.
11. Osgood, J. M. and Muraven, M. (2016). Does counting to ten increase or decrease aggression? The role of state self-control (ego-depletion) and consequences. *Journal of Applied Social Psychology, 46*(2), 105–13.
12. Lieberman, M. D., Eisenberger, N. I., Crockett, M. J., Tom, S. M., Pfeifer, J. H. and Way, B. M. (2007). Putting feelings into words. *Psychological Science, 18*(5), 421–8.
13. Sheppes, G. and Levin, Z. (2013). Emotion regulation choice: selecting between cognitive regulation strategies to control emotion. *Frontiers in Human Neuroscience, 7*, 179.
14. Gao, J., Fan, J., Wu, B. W., Halkias, G. T., Chau, M., Fung, P. C., ... and Sik, H. (2017). Repetitive religious chanting modulates the late-stage brain response to fear-and stress-provoking pictures. *Frontiers in Psychology, 7*, 2055.
15. Conrad, A. and Roth, W. T. (2007). Muscle relaxation therapy for anxiety disorders: it works but how? *Journal of Anxiety Disorders, 21*(3), 243–64.
16. Riskind, J. H. and Gotay, C. C. (1982). Physical posture: could it have regulatory or feedback effects on motivation and emotion? *Motivation and Emotion, 6*, 273–98.
17. Tsatsoulis, A. and Fountoulakis, S. (2006). The protective role of exercise on stress system dysregulation and comorbidities. *Annals of the New York Academy of Sciences, 1083*(1), 196–213.
18. Kinoshita, T., Nagata, S., Baba, R., Kohmoto, T. and Iwagaki, S. (2006). Cold-water face immersion per se elicits cardiac parasympathetic activity. *Circulation Journal, 70*(6), 773–6.
19. Albulescu, P., Macsinga, I., Sulea, C., Pap, Z., Tulbure, B. T. and Rusu, A. (2025). Short breaks during the workday and employee-related outcomes. A diary study. *Psychological Reports*, 00332941251317632.
20. Vøllestad, J., Nielsen, M. B. and Nielsen, G. H. (2012). Mindfulness- and acceptance-based interventions for anxiety disorders: a systematic review and meta-analysis. *British Journal of Clinical Psychology, 51*(3), 239–60.

Chapter 6

1. https://newsroom.accenture.com/news/2015/accenture-research-finds-listening-more-difficult-in-todays-digital-workplace
2. Ampaw-Farr, J. (2025). *Because of You, This is Me: The stories we tell, the stories we change and the power of everyday heroes.* Independent Thinking Press.
3. https://online.utpb.edu/about-us/articles/communication/how-much-of-communication-is-nonverbal/

4   Balban, M. Y., Cafaro, E., Saue-Fletcher, L., Washington, M. J., Bijanzadeh, M., Lee, A. M., ... and Huberman, A. D. (2021). Human responses to visually evoked threat. *Current Biology*, *31*(3), 601–12.

Chapter 7

1   https://menopausesupport.co.uk/?p=14434
2   Christianson, M. S., Ducie, J. A., Altman, K., Khafagy, A. M. and Shen, W. (2013). Menopause education: needs assessment of American obstetrics and gynecology residents. *Menopause*, *20*(11), 1120–5.
3   Cagnacci, A. and Venier, M. (2019). The controversial history of hormone replacement therapy. *Medicina*, *55*(9), 602.
4   https://www.nhs.uk/conditions/early-or-premature-menopause/
5   Harlow, S. D. and Paramsothy, P. (2011). Menstruation and the menopause transition. *Obstetrics and Gynecology Clinics of North America*, *38*(3), 595.
6   https://www.acog.org/womens-health/faqs/abnormal-uterine-bleeding
7   Scavello, I., Maseroli, E., Di Stasi, V. and Vignozzi, L. (2019). Sexual health in menopause. *Medicina*, *55*(9), 559.
8   https://www.nia.nih.gov/health/menopause/sex-and-menopause-treatment-symptoms
9   Newson, L. (2023). *The Definitive Guide to the Perimenopause and Menopause*. Yellow Kite; Newson, L. (2021). *Preparing for the Perimenopause and Menopause*. Yellow Kite.
10 https://www.newsonhealth.co.uk/newson-health-research/
11 https://www.balance-menopause.com/news/delayed-diagnosis-and-treatment-of-menopause-is-wasting-nhs-appointments-and-resources/
12 https://www.nice.org.uk/guidance/ng23
13 https://www.balance-menopause.com/news/delayed-diagnosis-and-treatment-of-menopause-is-wasting-nhs-appointments-and-resources/
14 Barber, K. and Charles, A. (2023). Barriers to accessing effective treatment and support for menopausal symptoms: a qualitative study capturing the behaviours, beliefs and experiences of key stakeholders. *Patient Preference and Adherence*, 2971–80.
15 Martin-Key, N. A., Funnell, E. L., Spadaro, B. and Bahn, S. (2023). Perceptions of healthcare provision throughout the menopause in the UK: a mixed-methods study. *NPJ Women's Health*, *1*(1), 2.
16 Quaile, H., O'Sullivan, A., Neville, A., Kamal, A., Glynne, S., Lewis, R., ... and Newson, L. (2025). Effect of HRT with and without testosterone on antidepressant deprescribing in perimenopausal and postmenopausal women with mood symptoms: a cross-sectional study. *The Journal of Sexual Medicine*, *22*(Supplement_1), qdaf068–081.
17 https://www.bma.org.uk/advice-and-support/nhs-delivery-and-workforce/pressures/nhs-backlog-data-analysis

18 Barber, K. and Charles, A. (2023). Barriers to accessing effective treatment and support for menopausal symptoms: a qualitative study capturing the behaviours, beliefs and experiences of key stakeholders. *Patient Preference and Adherence, 17*, 2971–80.
19 https://www.bma.org.uk/advice-and-support/gp-practices/managing-workload/general-practice-responsibility-in-responding-to-private-healthcare
20 https://www.theguardian.com/society/2019/may/21/gps-say-10-minute-appointment-with-doctor-is-too-short
21 https://pharmaceutical-journal.com/article/feature/is-hrt-overprescribed
22 https://www.newsonhealth.co.uk/pricing/
23 https://www.bma.org.uk/advice-and-support/gp-practices/managing-workload/general-practice-responsibility-in-responding-to-private-healthcare
24 Gajarawala, S. N. and Pelkowski, J. N. (2021). Telehealth benefits and barriers. *The Journal for Nurse Practitioners, 17*(2), 218–21.
25 Payne, R., Clarke, A., Swann, N., Van Dael, J., Brenman, N., Rosen, R., ... and Greenhalgh, T. (2024). Patient safety in remote primary care encounters: multimethod qualitative study combining Safety I and Safety II analysis. *BMJ Quality & Safety, 33*(9), 573–86.
26 Newson, L. and Rymer, J. (2019). The dangers of compounded bioidentical hormone replacement therapy. *The British Journal of General Practice, 69*(688), 540.
27 https://www.nhs.uk/conditions/menopause/treatment/
28 Panay, N. and Medical Advisory Council of the British Menopause Society (2019). BMS–Consensus statement: bioidentical HRT. *Post Reproductive Health, 25*(2), 61–3.
29 Peycheva, D., Wielgoszewska, B., Zaninotto, P., Steptoe, A. and Hardy, R. (2024). Employment trajectories during the menopause transition: experiences of women with early and surgical menopause. *medRxiv*, 2024–9.
30 https://www.royalfree.nhs.uk/patients-and-visitors/patient-information-leaflets/surgical-menopause
31 https://www.iapmd.org/surgery-surgical-menopause
32 https://www.cancerresearchuk.org/about-cancer/treatment/chemotherapy/fertility/womens-fertility-and-chemotherapy
33 https://www.macmillan.org.uk/cancer-information-and-support/treatment/types-of-treatment/radiotherapy/pelvic-radiotherapy/late-effects-of-pelvic-radiotherapy
34 Tang, H., Jia, Q., Dong, Z., Chen, Y., Shan, W., Wu, Y., ... and Chen, J. (2023). Add-back and combined regulation in GnRH-a treatment of endometriosis. *Clinical and Experimental Obstetrics & Gynecology, 50*(10), 224.

Chapter 8

1. https://www.nice.org.uk/news/articles/discussion-aid-to-support-clinical-conversations-about-hrt-published-alongside-updated-guidance
2. https://www.nhs.uk/conditions/menopause/treatment/
3. Ibid.
4. Harper-Harrison, G., Carlson, K. and Shanahan, M. M. (2024). Hormone replacement therapy. In *StatPearls* [Internet]. StatPearls Publishing.
5. https://www.nhs.uk/conditions/menopause/treatment/
6. https://www.nhs.uk/medicines/hormone-replacement-therapy-hrt/types-of-hormone-replacement-therapy-hrt/
7. Donovitz, G. S. (2022). A personal prospective on testosterone therapy in women: what we know in 2022. *Journal of Personalized Medicine, 12*(8), 1194.
8. Barber, K. and Charles, A. (2023). Barriers to accessing effective treatment and support for menopausal symptoms: a qualitative study capturing the behaviours, beliefs and experiences of key stakeholders. *Patient Preference and Adherence, 17*, 2971–80.
9. Ruan, X. and Mueck, A. O. (2022). Optimizing menopausal hormone therapy: for treatment and prevention, menstrual regulation, and reduction of possible risks. *Global Health Journal, 6*(2), 61–9.
10. Lippert, T. H., Mueck, A. O. and Seeger, H. (2000). Is the use of conjugated equine oestrogens in hormone replacement therapy still appropriate? *British Journal of Clinical Pharmacology, 49*(5), 489.
11. Files, J. A., Ko, M. G. and Pruthi, S. (2011, July). Bioidentical hormone therapy. *Mayo Clinic Proceedings, 86*(7), 673–80.
12. https://www.endocrine.org/patient-engagement/endocrine-library/hormones-and-endocrine-function/reproductive-hormones
13. Hariri, L. and Rehman, A. (2023). Estradiol (Updated 11 July 2022). StatPearls Publishing.
14. https://www.nhs.uk/medicines/hormone-replacement-therapy-hrt/types-of-hormone-replacement-therapy-hrt/
15. Ibid.
16. Ibid.
17. Harper-Harrison, G., Carlson, K. and Shanahan, M. M. (2024). Hormone replacement therapy. In *StatPearls* [Internet]. StatPearls Publishing.
18. https://www.chelwest.nhs.uk/your-visit/patient-leaflets/medicine-services/hormone-implants-in-hormone-replacement-therapy-hrt
19. Ibid.
20. https://www.nice.org.uk/guidance/ng23

21 https://www.endocrine.org/advocacy/position-statements/compounded-bioidentical-hormone-therapy
22 Newson, L. and Rymer, J. (2019). The dangers of compounded bioidentical hormone replacement therapy. *The British Journal of General Practice, 69*(688), 540.
23 Harper-Harrison, G., Carlson, K. and Shanahan, M. M. (2024). Hormone replacement therapy. In *StatPearls* [Internet]. StatPearls Publishing.
24 https://www.nhs.uk/conditions/menopause/treatment/
25 Ibid.
26 https://thebms.org.uk/publications/tools-for-clinicians/
27 https://www.nhs.uk/medicines/hormone-replacement-therapy-hrt/types-of-hormone-replacement-therapy-hrt/
28 Hirschberg, A. L. (2019). Hyperandrogenism in female athletes. *The Journal of Clinical Endocrinology & Metabolism, 104*(2), 503–5.
29 Uloko, M., Rahman, F., Puri, L. I. and Rubin, R. S. (2022). The clinical management of testosterone replacement therapy in postmenopausal women with hypoactive sexual desire disorder: a review. *International Journal of Impotence Research, 34*(7), 635–41.
30 https://www.health.harvard.edu/mens-health/treating-low-testosterone-levels
31 Guay, A., Munarriz, R., Jacobson, J., Talakoub, L., Traish, A., Quirk, F., ... and Spark, R. (2004). Serum androgen levels in healthy premenopausal women with and without sexual dysfunction: Part A. Serum androgen levels in women aged 20–49 years with no complaints of sexual dysfunction. *International Journal of Impotence Research, 16*(2), 112–20.
32 www.menopause.org.au/health-info/resources/testosterone-and-women
33 https://www.ashasexualhealth.org/hypoactive-sexual-desire-disorder/
34 Parish, S. J. and Kling, J. M. (2023). Testosterone use for hypoactive sexual desire disorder in postmenopausal women. *Menopause, 30*(7), 781–3.
35 Glaser, R. and Dimitrakakis, C. (2013). Testosterone therapy in women: myths and misconceptions. *Maturitas, 74*(3), 230–34.
36 https://www.nhs.uk/medicines/hormone-replacement-therapy-hrt/types-of-hormone-replacement-therapy-hrt/
37 https://www.fda.gov/drugs/postmarket-drug-safety-information-patients-and-providers/testosterone-information
38 https://www.nhs.uk/medicines/hormone-replacement-therapy-hrt/types-of-hormone-replacement-therapy-hrt/
39 Uloko, M., Rahman, F., Puri, L. I. and Rubin, R. S. (2022). The clinical management of testosterone replacement therapy in postmenopausal women with hypoactive sexual desire disorder: a review. *International Journal of Impotence Research, 34*(7), 635–41.

40 Glynne, S., Kamal, A., Kamel, A. M., Reisel, D. and Newson, L. (2025). Effect of transdermal testosterone therapy on mood and cognitive symptoms in peri-and postmenopausal women: a pilot study. *Archives of Women's Mental Health*, 28(3), 541–50.

41 Baik, S. H., Baye, F. and McDonald, C. J. (2024). Use of menopausal hormone therapy beyond age 65 years and its effects on women's health outcomes by types, routes, and doses. *Menopause*, 31(5), 363–75.

42 Newson Health (2024). *DLN Menopause Consumer Research: April 2024 Report*. Available at: https://www.newsonhealth.co.uk/wp-content/uploads/2024/10/DLN-Menopause-Consumer-Research-April-24-FINAL-Oct1.pdf

43 Hodis, H. N. and Mack, W. J. (2022). Menopausal hormone replacement therapy and reduction of all-cause mortality and cardiovascular disease: it is about time and timing. *The Cancer Journal*, 28(3), 208–23.

44 Maki, P. M. (2013). Critical window hypothesis of hormone therapy and cognition: a scientific update on clinical studies. *Menopause*, 20(6), 695–709.

45 Gambacciani, M. and Levancini, M. (2014). Hormone replacement therapy and the prevention of postmenopausal osteoporosis. *Menopause Review/Przegląd Menopauzalny*, 13(4), 213–20.

46 https://www.nhs.uk/medicines/hormone-replacement-therapy-hrt/benefits-and-risks-of-hormone-replacement-therapy-hrt/

47 Abdi, F., Mobedi, H., Bayat, F., Mosaffa, N., Dolatian, M. and Tehrani, F. R. (2017). The effects of transdermal estrogen delivery on bone mineral density in postmenopausal women: a meta-analysis. *Iranian Journal of Pharmaceutical Research: IJPR*, 16(1), 380.

48 Hodis, H. N. and Mack, W. J. (2022). Menopausal hormone replacement therapy and reduction of all-cause mortality and cardiovascular disease: it is about time and timing. *The Cancer Journal*, 28(3), 208–23.

49 Nerattini, M., Jett, S., Andy, C., Carlton, C., Zarate, C., Boneu, C., ... and Mosconi, L. (2023). Systematic review and meta-analysis of the effects of menopause hormone therapy on risk of Alzheimer's disease and dementia. *Frontiers in Aging Neuroscience*, 15, 1260427.

50 Shih, Y. H., Yang, C. Y., Wang, S. J. and Lung, C. C. (2024). Menopausal hormone therapy decreases the likelihood of diabetes development in peri-menopausal individuals with prediabetes. *Diabetes & Metabolism*, 50(4), 101546.

51 Labadie, J. D., Harrison, T. A., Banbury, B., Amtay, E. L., Bernd, S., Brenner, H., ... and Newcomb, P. A. (2020). Postmenopausal hormone therapy and colorectal cancer risk by molecularly defined subtypes and tumor location. *JNCI Cancer Spectrum*, 4(5), pkaa042.

52 Holroyd, C. R. and Edwards, C. J. (2009). The effects of hormone replacement therapy on autoimmune disease: rheumatoid arthritis and systemic lupus erythematosus. *Climacteric, 12*(5), 378–86.
53 Glynne, S., Kamal, A., McColl, L., Newson, L., Reisel, D., Mu, E., ... and Kulkarni, J. (2025). Transdermal oestradiol and testosterone therapy for menopausal depression and mood symptoms: retrospective cohort study. *The British Journal of Psychiatry, 16*, 1–10.
54 Barber, K. and Charles, A. (2023). Barriers to accessing effective treatment and support for menopausal symptoms: a qualitative study capturing the behaviours, beliefs and experiences of key stakeholders. *Patient Preference and Adherence, 17*, 2971–80.
55 Stute, P., Marsden, J., Salih, N. and Cagnacci, A. (2023). Reappraising 21 years of the WHI study: putting the findings in context for clinical practice. *Maturitas, 174*, 8–13.
56 https://www.nhs.uk/medicines/hormone-replacement-therapy-hrt/benefits-and-risks-of-hormone-replacement-therapy-hrt/
57 Crawford, S. L., Crandall, C. J., Derby, C. A., El Khoudary, S. R., Waetjen, L. E., Fischer, M. and Joffe, H. (2019). Menopausal hormone therapy trends before versus after 2002: impact of the Women's Health Initiative Study Results. *Menopause, 26*(6), 588–97.
58 Miller, V. M. and Manson, J. E. (2013). Women's health initiative hormone therapy trials: new insights on cardiovascular disease from additional years of follow up. *Current Cardiovascular Risk Reports, 7*, 196–202.
59 Rossouw, J. E., Anderson, G. L., Prentice, R. L., LaCroix, A. Z., Kooperberg, C., Stefanick, M. L., ... and Ockene, J. (2002). Risks and benefits of estrogen plus progestin in healthy postmenopausal women: principal results from the Women's Health Initiative randomized controlled trial. *Jama, 288*(3), 321–33.
60 Rossouw, J. E., Anderson, G. L., Prentice, R. L., LaCroix, A. Z., Kooperberg, C., Stefanick, M. L., ... and Ockene, J. (2002). Risks and benefits of estrogen plus progestin in healthy postmenopausal women: principal results from the Women's Health Initiative randomized controlled trial. *Jama, 288*(3), 321–33.
61 Hodis, H. N. and Mack, W. J. (2022). Menopausal hormone replacement therapy and reduction of all-cause mortality and cardiovascular disease: it is about time and timing. *The Cancer Journal, 28*(3), 208–23.
62 Barber, K. and Charles, A. (2023). Barriers to accessing effective treatment and support for menopausal symptoms: a qualitative study capturing the behaviours, beliefs and experiences of key stakeholders. *Patient Preference and Adherence, 17*, 2971–80.

63 Fournier, A., Berrino, F., Riboli, E., Avenel, V. and Clavel-Chapelon, F. (2005). Breast cancer risk in relation to different types of hormone replacement therapy in the E3N-EPIC cohort. *International Journal of Cancer, 114*(3), 448–54.
64 Vinogradova, Y., Coupland, C. and Hippisley-Cox, J. (2020). Use of hormone replacement therapy and risk of breast cancer: nested case-control studies using the QResearch and CPRD databases. *British Medical Journal, 371*.
65 Ibid.
66 Ibid.
67 Nahmias-Blank, D., Maimon, O., Meirovitz, A., Sheva, K., Peretz-Yablonski, T. and Elkin, M. (2023, November). Excess body weight and postmenopausal breast cancer: emerging molecular mechanisms and perspectives. *Seminars in Cancer Biology, 96,* 26–35.
68 https://www.cancer.org/cancer/types/breast-cancer/risk-and-prevention/lifestyle-related-breast-cancer-risk-factors.html
69 https://www.komen.org/breast-cancer/risk-factor/smoking/
70 Lee, J., Lee, J., Lee, D. W., Kim, H. R. and Kang, M. Y. (2021). Sedentary work and breast cancer risk: a systematic review and meta-analysis. *Journal of Occupational Health, 63*(1), e12239.
71 https://www.nhs.uk/medicines/hormone-replacement-therapy-hrt/benefits-and-risks-of-hormone-replacement-therapy-hrt/
72 The Menopause Charity (2021). *The myths vs the facts* [Fact sheet]. Retrieved from https://www.themenopausecharity.org/wp-content/uploads/2021/04/The-myths-vs-the-facts-.pdf
73 Mawet, M., Gaspard, U. and Foidart, J. M. (2021). Estetrol as estrogen in a combined oral contraceptive, from the first in-human study to the contraceptive efficacy. *European Journal of Gynecology and Obstetrics, 3*(1), 3–21.
74 https://www.nhs.uk/medicines/sildenafil-viagra/side-effects-of-sildenafil/
75 Monroe, K. R., Stanczyk, F. Z., Besinque, K. H. and Pike, M. C. (2013). The effect of grapefruit intake on endogenous serum estrogen levels in postmenopausal women. *Nutrition and Cancer, 65*(5), 644–52.
76 https://www.nhs.uk/medicines/hormone-replacement-therapy-hrt/continuous-combined-hormone-replacement-therapy-hrt-tablets-capsules-and-patches/taking-continuous-combined-hrt-with-other-medicines-and-herbal-supplements/
77 Ibid.
78 Pinkerton, J. A., Aguirre, F. S., Blake, J., Cosman, F., Hodis, H., Hoffstetter, S., … and Utian, W. H. (2017). The 2017 hormone therapy position statement of the North American Menopause Society. *Menopause: The Journal of the North American Menopause Society,* 728–53.

79 Wang, X. J. (2024). Research status of hormone replacement therapy on mood and sleep quality in menopausal women. *World Journal of Psychiatry*, *14*(9), 1289.
80 https://www.nice.org.uk/guidance/qs143/chapter/quality-statement-1-diagnosing-perimenopause-and-menopause
81 https://academic.oup.com/jcem/article/100/11/3975/2836060
82 Marjoribanks, J., Farquhar, C., Roberts, H. and Lethaby, A. (2012). Long-term hormone therapy for perimenopausal and postmenopausal women. *Cochrane Database of Systematic Reviews*, *1*(1), CD004143.
83 Lethaby, A., Marjoribanks, J., Kronenberg, F., Roberts, H., Eden, J. and Brown, J. (2013). Phytoestrogens for menopausal vasomotor symptoms. *Cochrane Database of Systematic Reviews*, (12), CD001395.
84 https://www.nhs.uk/medicines/hormone-replacement-therapy-hrt/when-to-take-hormone-replacement-therapy-hrt/
85 https://www.gov.uk/government/publications/glp-1-medicines-for-weight-loss-and-diabetes-what-you-need-to-know/glp-1-medicines-for-weight-loss-and-diabetes-what-you-need-to-know
86 Neeland, I. J., Linge, J. and Birkenfeld, A. L. (2024). Changes in lean body mass with glucagon-like peptide-1-based therapies and mitigation strategies. *Diabetes, Obesity and Metabolism*, *26*, 16–27.
87 https://thebms.org.uk/2025/04/new-bms-tool-for-clinicians-use-of-incretin-based-therapies-in-women-using-hrt/
88 https://www.gov.uk/government/publications/glp-1-medicines-for-weight-loss-and-diabetes-what-you-need-to-know/glp-1-medicines-for-weight-loss-and-diabetes-what-you-need-to-know
89 British Menopause Society (2025). Use of incretin-based therapies (e.g. GLP-1 receptor agonists) in women around the time of menopause: a BMS toolkit for clinicians. Available at: https://thebms.org.uk/wp-content/uploads/2025/05/23-BMS-TfC-Use-of-incretin-based-therapies-APRIL2025-E.pdf
90 https://www.gov.uk/government/news/mhra-warns-of-unsafe-fake-weight-loss-pens
91 https://www.nhs.uk/medicines/hormone-replacement-therapy-hrt/side-effects-of-hormone-replacement-therapy-hrt/
92 https://www.nhs.uk/medicines/hormone-replacement-therapy-hrt/oestrogen-tablets-patches-gel-and-spray/side-effects-of-oestrogen-tablets-patches-gel-and-spray/
93 https://www.nhs.uk/medicines/hormone-replacement-therapy-hrt/when-to-take-hormone-replacement-therapy-hrt/
94 Muir, K. (2022). *Everything You Need to Know about the Menopause (But Were Too Afraid to Ask)*. Simon & Schuster UK.

95 https://www.nhs.uk/medicines/hormone-replacement-therapy-hrt/continuous-combined-hormone-replacement-therapy-hrt-tablets-capsules-and-patches/who-can-and-cannot-take-continuous-combined-hrt/
96 Barber, K. and Charles, A. (2023). Barriers to accessing effective treatment and support for menopausal symptoms: a qualitative study capturing the behaviours, beliefs and experiences of key stakeholders. *Patient Preference and Adherence*, *17*, 2971–80.
97 Dahlgren, M. K., Kosereisoglu, D., Smith, R. T., Sagar, K. A., Lambros, A. M., El-Abboud, C. and Gruber, S. A. (2023). Identifying variables associated with menopause-related shame and stigma: results from a national survey study. *Journal of Women's Health*, *32*(11), 1182–91.
98 Newhouser, L. M., Maneval, M., Rayalam, K., Sabeeh, G. and Varela, L. (2022). SSRIs vs. SNRIs for vasomotor symptoms of menopause. *American Family Physician*, *105*(4), 430–31.
99 Johnson, E. D. and Carroll, D. G. (2011). Venlafaxine and desvenlafaxine in the management of menopausal hot flashes. *Pharmacy Practice*, *9*(3), 117.
100 https://www.nhs.uk/medicines/hormone-replacement-therapy-hrt/alternatives-to-hormone-replacement-therapy-hrt/other-medicines-for-menopause-symptoms/
101 Archer, C., Wiles, N., Kessler, D., Turner, K. and Caldwell, D. M. (2024). Beta-blockers for the treatment of anxiety disorders: a systematic review and meta-analysis. *Journal of Affective Disorders*, *368*, 90–9.
102 https://www.healthline.com/health/menopause/symptoms-of-menopause-while-on-birth-control-pills
103 https://www.nhs.uk/contraception/methods-of-contraception/combined-pill/who-can-take-it/
104 https://www.nhs.uk/medicines/hormone-replacement-therapy-hrt/types-of-hormone-replacement-therapy-hrt/
105 https://www.nhs.uk/contraception/methods-of-contraception/ius-hormonal-coil/what-is-it/
106 https://www.nhs.uk/contraception/methods-of-contraception/ius-hormonal-coil/side-effects-and-risks/
107 https://www.nhs.uk/contraception/methods-of-contraception/ius-hormonal-coil/getting-it-fitted-or-removed/
108 Freedman, R. R. and Dinsay, R. (2000). Clonidine raises the sweating threshold in symptomatic but not in asymptomatic postmenopausal women. *Fertility and Sterility*, *74*(1), 20–3.
109 https://www.nhs.uk/medicines/hormone-replacement-therapy-hrt/alternatives-to-hormone-replacement-therapy-hrt/other-medicines-for-menopause-symptoms/

110 Allameh, Z., Rouholamin, S. and Valaie, S. (2013). Comparison of gabapentin with estrogen for treatment of hot flashes in post-menopausal women. *Journal of Research in Pharmacy Practice*, 2(2), 64–9.
111 Yoon, S. H., Lee, J. Y., Lee, C., Lee, H. and Kim, S. N. (2020). Gabapentin for the treatment of hot flushes in menopause: a meta-analysis. *Menopause*, 27(4), 485–93.
112 https://www.nice.org.uk/guidance/ng23
113 https://www.nice.org.uk/guidance/ng23/chapter/recommendations
114 Borud, E. K., Alraek, T., White, A., Fonnebo, V., Eggen, A. E., Hammar, M., ... and Grimsgaard, S. (2009). The acupuncture on hot flushes among menopausal women (ACUFLASH) study, a randomized controlled trial. *Menopause*, 16(3), 484–93.
115 Susanti, H. D., Sonko, I., Chang, P. C., Chuang, Y. H. and Chung, M. H. (2022). Effects of yoga on menopausal symptoms and sleep quality across menopause statuses: a randomized controlled trial. *Nursing & Health Sciences*, 24(2), 368–79.
116 https://www.nhs.uk/medicines/hormone-replacement-therapy-hrt/alternatives-to-hormone-replacement-therapy-hrt/herbal-remedies-and-complementary-medicines-for-menopause-symptoms/
117 https://www.nhs.uk/tests-and-treatments/herbal-medicines/
118 Kaye, P. (2024). *The Science of Menopause: Understand Your Body, Make the Right Choices*. Dorling Kindersley.

Chapter 9

1 Women's Health Concern (2023). Weight gain and menopause: a factsheet for women. Available at: https://www.womens-health-concern.org/wp-content/uploads/2023/06/31-WHC-FACTSHEET-Weight-Gain-and-menopause-JUNE2023-A.pdf
2 Ibid.
3 Lovejoy, J. C., Champagne, C. M., De Jonge, L., Xie, H. and Smith, S. R. (2008). Increased visceral fat and decreased energy expenditure during the menopausal transition. *International Journal of Obesity*, 32(6), 949–58.
4 Dal Brun, D., Pescarini, E., Calonaci, S., Bonello, E. and Meneguzzo, P. (2024). Body evaluation in men: the role of body weight dissatisfaction in appearance evaluation, eating, and muscle dysmorphia psychopathology. *Journal of Eating Disorders*, 12(1), 65.
5 https://www.ucl.ac.uk/news/2021/jan/fifth-adults-have-mental-health-problems-midlife
6 Gondek, D., Bernardi, L., McElroy, E. and Comolli, C. L. (2024). Why do middle-aged adults report worse mental health and wellbeing than younger adults? An exploratory network analysis of the Swiss Household Panel data. *Applied Research in Quality of Life*, 19(4), 1459–500.

References

7. Ng, M., Dai, X., Cogen, R. M., Abdelmasseh, M., Abdollahi, A., Abdullahi, A., ... and Khan, M. S. (2024). National-level and state-level prevalence of overweight and obesity among children, adolescents, and adults in the USA, 1990–2021, and forecasts up to 2050. *The Lancet*, *404*(10469), 2278–98; https://digital.nhs.uk/data-and-information/publications/statistical/statistics-on-obesity-physical-activity-and-diet/england-2021
8. Roh, E. and Choi, K. M. (2020). Health consequences of sarcopenic obesity: a narrative review. *Frontiers in Endocrinology*, *11*, 332.
9. Pelusi, C. and Pasquali, R. (2012). The significance of low testosterone levels in obese men. *Current Obesity Reports*, *1*, 181–90.
10. Rojas-Zambrano, J. G., Rojas-Zambrano, A., Rojas-Zambrano, A. F. and Rojas-Zambrano Sr, A. F. (2025). Impact of testosterone on male health: a systematic review. *Cureus*, *17*(4).
11. Janssen, I., Katzmarzyk, P. T. and Ross, R. (2002). Body mass index, waist circumference, and health risk: evidence in support of current National Institutes of Health guidelines. *Archives of Internal Medicine*, *162*(18), 2074–9.
12. Li, Y., He, H., Wang, J., Chen, Y., Wang, C., Li, X., ... and Lei, X. (2023). Effect of multidisciplinary health education based on lifestyle medicine on menopausal syndrome and lifestyle behaviors of menopausal women: a clinical controlled study. *Frontiers in Public Health*, *11*, 1119352.
13. Zapalac, K., Miller, M., Champagne, F. A., Schnyer, D. M. and Baird, B. (2024). The effects of physical activity on sleep architecture and mood in naturalistic environments. *Scientific Reports*, *14*(1), 5637.
14. Park, J. H., Moon, J. H., Kim, H. J., Kong, M. H. and Oh, Y. H. (2020). Sedentary lifestyle: overview of updated evidence of potential health risks. *Korean Journal of Family Medicine*, *41*(6), 365.
15. Akash, M. S. and Chowdhury, S. (2025). Small changes, big impact: a mini review of habit formation and behavioral change principles. *World Journal of Advanced Research and Reviews*, *26*(1), 3098–106.
16. Woods, N. F., Mitchell, E. S. and Smith-DiJulio, K. (2009). Cortisol levels during the menopausal transition and early postmenopause: observations from the Seattle Midlife Women's Health Study. *Menopause*, *16*(4), 708–18; Kuck, M. J. and Hogervorst, E. (2024). Stress, depression, and anxiety: psychological complaints across menopausal stages. *Frontiers in Psychiatry*, *15*, 1323743.
17. Mental Health UK (2025). *The Burnout Report 2025*. Available at: https://euc7zxtct58.exactdn.com/wp-content/uploads/2025/01/16142505/Mental-Health-UK_The-Burnout-Report-2025.pdf
18. Ibid.

19 https://www.apa.org/pubs/reports/work-in-america/2023-workplace-health-well-being
20 Kuck, M. J. and Hogervorst, E. (2024). Stress, depression, and anxiety: psychological complaints across menopausal stages. *Frontiers in Psychiatry*, *15*, 1323743.
21 Turek, J. and Gąsior, Ł. (2023). Estrogen fluctuations during the menopausal transition are a risk factor for depressive disorders. *Pharmacological Reports*, *75*(1), 32–43.
22 Mitchell, E. S. and Woods, N. F. (2015). Hot flush severity during the menopausal transition and early postmenopause: beyond hormones. *Climacteric*, *18*(4), 536–44.
23 Chu, B., Marwaha, K., Sanvictores, T., Awosika, A. O. and Ayers, D. (2024). Physiology, stress reaction. In *StatPearls* [Internet]. StatPearls Publishing.
24 Goldfarb, E. V. (2019). Enhancing memory with stress: progress, challenges, and opportunities. *Brain and Cognition*, *133*, 94–105.
25 https://www.mayoclinic.org/healthy-lifestyle/stress-management/in-depth/stress/art-20046037
26 Kuck, M. J. and Hogervorst, E. (2024). Stress, depression, and anxiety: psychological complaints across menopausal stages. *Frontiers in Psychiatry*, *15*, 1323743.
27 Chu, B., Marwaha, K., Sanvictores, T., Awosika, A. O. and Ayers, D. (2024). Physiology, stress reaction. In *StatPearls* [Internet]. StatPearls Publishing.
28 https://www.apa.org/topics/stress/body
29 Herman, J. P., McKlveen, J. M., Ghosal, S., Kopp, B., Wulsin, A., Makinson, R., ... and Myers, B. (2016). Regulation of the hypothalamic-pituitary-adrenocortical stress response. *Comprehensive Physiology*, *6*(2), 603.
30 https://www.yourhormones.info/hormones/cortisol/
31 Kumari, M., Badrick, E., Chandola, T., Adam, E. K., Stafford, M., Marmot, M. G., ... and Kivimaki, M. (2009). Cortisol secretion and fatigue: associations in a community-based cohort. *Psychoneuroendocrinology*, *34*(10), 1476–85.
32 https://news.yale.edu/2000/09/22/stress-may-cause-excess-abdominal-fat-otherwise-slender-women-study-conducted-yale-shows
33 Alotiby, A. (2024). Immunology of stress: a review article. *Journal of Clinical Medicine*, *13*(21), 6394.
34 Gecaite-Stonciene, J., Hughes, B. M., Kazukauskiene, N., Bunevicius, A., Burkauskas, J., Neverauskas, J., ... and Mickuviene, N. (2022). Cortisol response to psychosocial stress, mental distress, fatigue and quality of life in coronary artery disease patients. *Scientific Reports*, *12*(1), 19373.
35 Echouffo-Tcheugui, J. B., Conner, S. C., Himali, J. J., Maillard, P., DeCarli, C. S., Beiser, A. S., ... and Seshadri, S. (2018). Circulating cortisol

and cognitive and structural brain measures: The Framingham Heart Study. *Neurology*, *91*(21), e1961–70.
36 Passos, G. S., Youngstedt, S. D., Rozales, A. A. R. C., Ferreira, W. S., De-Assis, D. E., De-Assis, B. P. and Santana, M. G. (2023). Insomnia severity is associated with morning cortisol and psychological health. *Sleep Science*, *16*(01), 92–6.
37 https://www.endocrine.org/patient-engagement/endocrine-library/hormones-and-endocrine-function/adrenal-hormones
38 https://www.endocrine.org/patient-engagement/endocrine-library/hormones-and-endocrine-function/adrenal-hormones
39 Morilak, D. A., Barrera, G., Echevarria, D. J., Garcia, A. S., Hernandez, A., Ma, S. and Petre, C. O. (2005). Role of brain norepinephrine in the behavioral response to stress. *Progress in Neuro-psychopharmacology and Biological Psychiatry*, *29*(8), 1214–24.
40 https://www.endocrine.org/patient-engagement/endocrine-library/hormones-and-endocrine-function/adrenal-hormones
41 Cui, J., Li, M., Wei, Y., Li, H., He, X., Yang, Q., ... and Qin, D. (2022). Inhalation aromatherapy via brain-targeted nasal delivery: natural volatiles or essential oils on mood disorders. *Frontiers in Pharmacology*, *13*, 860043.
42 https://www.apa.org/ptsd-guideline/patients-and-families/cognitive-behavioral
43 Walker, J., Muench, A., Perlis, M. L. and Vargas, I. (2022). Cognitive behavioral
therapy for insomnia (CBT-I): a primer. *Klinicheskaia i spetsial'naia psikhologiia / Clinical Psychology and Special Education*, *11*(2), 123.
44 https://pubmed.ncbi.nlm.nih.gov/36908717/
45 Fincham, G. W., Strauss, C., Montero-Marin, J. and Cavanagh, K. (2023). Effect of breathwork on stress and mental health: a meta-analysis of randomised-controlled trials. *Scientific Reports*, *13*(1), 432.
46 Ma, X., Yue, Z. Q., Gong, Z. Q., Zhang, H., Duan, N. Y., Shi, Y. T., ... and Li, Y. F. (2017). The effect of diaphragmatic breathing on attention, negative affect and stress in healthy adults. *Frontiers in Psychology*, *8*, 234806.
47 Balban, M. Y., Neri, E., Kogon, M. M., Weed, L., Nouriani, B., Jo, B., ... and Huberman, A. D. (2023). Brief structured respiration practices enhance mood and reduce physiological arousal. *Cell Reports Medicine*, *4*(1).
48 Smyth, J. M., Johnson, J. A., Auer, B. J., Lehman, E., Talamo, G. and Sciamanna, C. N. (2018). Online positive affect journaling in the improvement of mental distress and well-being in general medical patients with elevated anxiety symptoms: a preliminary randomized controlled trial. *JMIR mental health*, *5*(4), e11290.
49 Basso, J. C., McHale, A., Ende, V., Oberlin, D. J. and Suzuki, W. A. (2019). Brief, daily meditation enhances attention, memory, mood, and

emotional regulation in non-experienced meditators. *Behavioural Brain Research*, *356*, 208–20.

50 Hoge, E. A., Bui, E., Marques, L., Metcalf, C. A., Morris, L. K., Robinaugh, D. J., ... and Simon, N. M. (2013). Randomized controlled trial of mindfulness meditation for generalized anxiety disorder: effects on anxiety and stress reactivity. *The Journal of Clinical Psychiatry*, *74*(8), 16662.

51 Simon, K. C., McDevitt, E. A., Ragano, R. and Mednick, S. C. (2022). Progressive muscle relaxation increases slow-wave sleep during a daytime nap. *Journal of Sleep Research*, *31*(5), e13574.

52 Lo Martire, V., Berteotti, C., Zoccoli, G. and Bastianini, S. (2024). Improving sleep to improve stress resilience. *Current Sleep Medicine Reports*, *10*(1), 23–33.

53 Acoba, E. F. (2024). Social support and mental health: the mediating role of perceived stress. *Frontiers in Psychology*, *15*, 1330720.

54 Albulescu, P., Macsinga, I., Rusu, A., Sulea, C., Bodnaru, A. and Tulbure, B. T. (2022). 'Give me a break!' A systematic review and meta-analysis on the efficacy of micro-breaks for increasing well-being and performance. *PlOS One*, *17*(8), e0272460.

55 Martire, V. L., Caruso, D., Palagini, L., Zoccoli, G. and Bastianini, S. (2020). Stress & sleep: a relationship lasting a lifetime. *Neuroscience & Biobehavioral Reviews*, *117*, 65–77.

56 Tomaso, C. C., Johnson, A. B. and Nelson, T. D. (2021). The effect of sleep deprivation and restriction on mood, emotion, and emotion regulation: three meta-analyses in one. *Sleep*, *44*(6), zsaa289.

57 Troìa, L., Garassino, M., Volpicelli, A. I., Fornara, A., Libretti, A., Surico, D. and Remorgida, V. (2025). Sleep disturbance and perimenopause: a narrative review. *Journal of Clinical Medicine*, *14*(5), 1479.

58 Joffe, H., Massler, A. and Sharkey, K. M. (2010, September). Evaluation and management of sleep disturbance during the menopause transition. *Seminars in Reproductive Medicine*, *28*(5), 404–21. Thieme Medical Publishers.

59 https://www.ninds.nih.gov/health-information/public-education/brain-basics/brain-basics-understanding-sleep

60 https://www.ninds.nih.gov/health-information/public-education/brain-basics/brain-basics-understanding-sleep

61 Chaput, J. P., McHill, A. W., Cox, R. C., Broussard, J. L., Dutil, C., da Costa, B. G., ... and Wright Jr, K. P. (2023). The role of insufficient sleep and circadian misalignment in obesity. *Nature Reviews Endocrinology*, *19*(2), 82–97.

62 https://www.froedtert.com/stories/sleep-deprivation-effects-symptoms-and-causes

63 Watson, N. F., Badr, M. S., Belenky, G. and Bliwise, D. L. Buxton. OM, Buysee, D.,... and Tasali, E. (2015). Recommended amount of sleep for a healthy adult: a joint consensus statement of the American Academy of Sleep Medicine and Sleep Research Society. *Sleep*, *38*(6), 843–4.

64 Hein, E., Halonen, R., Wolbers, T., Makkonen, T., Kyllönen, M., Kuula, L., ... and Pesonen, A. K. (2024). Does sleep promote adaptation to acute stress: An experimental study. *Neurobiology of stress*, *29*, 100613.

65 Vitale, K. C., Owens, R., Hopkins, S. R. and Malhotra, A. (2019). Sleep hygiene for optimizing recovery in athletes: review and recommendations. *International Journal of Sports Nedicine*, *40*(08), 535–543.

66 Medic, G., Wille, M. and Hemels, M. E. (2017). Short-and long-term health consequences of sleep disruption. *Nature and Science of Sleep*, 151–61.

67 Gardiner, C., Weakley, J., Burke, L. M., Roach, G. D., Sargent, C., Maniar, N., ... and Halson, S. L. (2023). The effect of caffeine on subsequent sleep: a systematic review and meta-analysis. *Sleep Medicine Reviews*, *69*, 101764.

68 Baron, K. G., Abbott, S., Jao, N., Manalo, N. and Mullen, R. (2017). Orthosomnia: are some patients taking the quantified self too far? *Journal of Clinical Sleep Medicine*, *13*(2), 351–4.

69 Mukherjee, U., Sehar, U., Brownell, M. and Reddy, P. H. (2024). Sleep deprivation in dementia comorbidities: Focus on cardiovascular disease, diabetes, anxiety/depression and thyroid disorders. *Aging*, *16*(21), 13409; Ungvari, Z., Fekete, M., Lehoczki, A., Munkácsy, G., Fekete, J. T., Zábó, V., ... and Győrffy, B. (2025). Sleep disorders increase the risk of dementia, Alzheimer's disease, and cognitive decline: a meta-analysis. *GeroScience*, 1–22.

70 Anderson, A. R., Ostermiller, L., Lastrapes, M. and Hales, L. (2025). Does sunlight exposure predict next-night sleep? A daily diary study among US adults. *Journal of Health Psychology*, *30*(5), 962–75.

71 Hjetland, G. J., Skogen, J. C., Hysing, M., Gradisar, M. and Sivertsen, B. (2025). How and when screens are used: comparing different screen activities and sleep in Norwegian university students. *Frontiers in Psychiatry*, *16*, 1548273.

72 Okamoto-Mizuno, K. and Mizuno, K. (2012). Effects of thermal environment on sleep and circadian rhythm. *Journal of Physiological Anthropology*, *31*, 1–9.

73 Chaput, J. P., Dutil, C., Featherstone, R., Ross, R., Giangregorio, L., Saunders, T. J., ... and Carrier, J. (2020). Sleep timing, sleep consistency, and health in adults: a systematic review. *Applied Physiology, Nutrition, and Metabolism*, *45*(10), S232–S247.

74 Åkerstedt, T., Orsini, N., Petersen, H., Axelsson, J., Lekander, M. and Kecklund, G. (2012). Predicting sleep quality from stress and prior

sleep – a study of day-to-day covariation across six weeks. *Sleep Medicine, 13*(6), 674–9.
75 Lastella, M., Miller, D. J., Montero, A., Sprajcer, M., Ferguson, S. A., Browne, M. and Vincent, G. E. (2025). Sleep on it: a pilot study exploring the impact of sexual activity on sleep outcomes in cohabiting couples. *Sleep Health, 11*(2), 198–205.
76 Ibid.
77 Qaseem, A., Kansagara, D., Forciea, M. A., Cooke, M., Denberg, T. D. and Clinical Guidelines Committee of the American College of Physicians (2016). Management of chronic insomnia disorder in adults: a clinical practice guideline from the American College of Physicians. *Annals of Internal Medicine, 165*(2), 125–33.
78 Kalmbach, D. A., Cheng, P., Arnedt, J. T., Cuamatzi-Castelan, A., Atkinson, R. L., Fellman-Couture, C., ... and Drake, C. L. (2019). Improving daytime functioning, work performance, and quality of life in postmenopausal women with insomnia: comparing cognitive behavioral therapy for insomnia, sleep restriction therapy, and sleep hygiene education. *Journal of Clinical Sleep Medicine, 15*(7), 999–1010.
79 Morin, C. M., Bootzin, R. R., Buysse, D. J., Edinger, J. D., Espie, C. A. and Lichstein, K. L. (2006). Psychological and behavioral treatment of insomnia: update of the recent evidence (1998–2004). *Sleep, 29*(11), 1398–414.
80 Baldwin, D. S. and Papakostas, G. I. (2006). Symptoms of fatigue and sleepiness in major depressive disorder. *Journal of Clinical Psychiatry, 67*, 9.
81 Gardiner, C., Weakley, J., Burke, L. M., Roach, G. D., Sargent, C., Maniar, N., ... and Halson, S. L. (2023). The effect of caffeine on subsequent sleep: a systematic review and meta-analysis. *Sleep Medicine Reviews, 69*, 101764.
82 Reichert, C. F., Deboer, T. and Landolt, H. P. (2022). Adenosine, caffeine, and sleep–wake regulation: state of the science and perspectives. *Journal of Sleep Research, 31*(4), e13597; Thölke, P., Arcand-Lavigne, M., Lajnef, T., Frenette, S., Carrier, J. and Jerbi, K. (2025). Caffeine induces age-dependent increases in brain complexity and criticality during sleep. *Communications Biology, 8*(1), 685.
83 McCullar, K. S., Barker, D. H., McGeary, J. E., Saletin, J. M., Gredvig-Ardito, C., Swift, R. M. and Carskadon, M. A. (2024). Altered sleep architecture following consecutive nights of presleep alcohol. *Sleep, 47*(4), zsae003.
84 Angarita, G. A., Emadi, N., Hodges, S. and Morgan, P. T. (2016). Sleep abnormalities associated with alcohol, cannabis, cocaine, and opiate use: a comprehensive review. *Addiction Science & Clinical Practice, 11*, 1–17.

85 https://www.sleepfoundation.org/sleep-hygiene/scandinavian-sleep-method
86 Li, X., Halaki, M. and Chow, C. M. (2024). How do sleepwear and bedding fibre types affect sleep quality? A systematic review. *Journal of Sleep Research*, *33*(6), e14217.
87 Testa, D. and Stoikovitch, D. (2022). A thermoregulated pillow improves sleep: results from real-life data. *SLEEP*, *45*, A37–8.
88 Avis, N. E., Levine, B. J. and Coeytaux, R. (2022). Results of a pilot study of a cooling mattress pad to reduce vasomotor symptoms and improve sleep. *Menopause*, *29*(8), 973–8.
89 Ibid.
90 Park, H., Parker, G. L., Boardman, C. H., Morris, M. M. and Smith, T. J. (2011). A pilot phase II trial of magnesium supplements to reduce menopausal hot flashes in breast cancer patients. *Supportive Care in Cancer*, *19*, 859–63.
91 Dutheil, F., Danini, B., Bagheri, R., Fantini, M. L., Pereira, B., Moustafa, F., ... and Navel, V. (2021). Effects of a short daytime nap on the cognitive performance: a systematic review and meta-analysis. *International Journal of Environmental Research and Public Health*, *18*(19), 10212.
92 Wofford, N., Ceballos, N., Elkins, G. and Westerberg, C. E. (2022). A brief nap during an acute stressor improves negative affect. *Journal of Sleep Research*, *31*(6), e13701.
93 Vizmanos, B., Cascales, A. I., Rodríguez-Martín, M., Salmerón, D., Morales, E., Aragón-Alonso, A., ... and Garaulet, M. (2023). Lifestyle mediators of associations among siestas, obesity, and metabolic health. *Obesity*, *31*(5), 1227–39.
94 Oriyama, S. (2023). Effects of 90- and 30-min naps or a 120-min nap on alertness and performance: reanalysis of an existing pilot study. *Scientific Reports*, *13*(1), 9862.
95 Mograss, M., Abi-Jaoude, J., Frimpong, E., Chalati, D., Moretto, U., Tarelli, L., ... and Dang-Vu, T. T. (2022). The effects of napping on night-time sleep in healthy young adults. *Journal of Sleep Research*, *31*(5), e13578.
96 Littlehales, N. (2016). *Sleep: The Myth of 8 Hours, the Power of Naps … and the New Plan to Recharge Your Body and Mind*. Penguin Life.

Chapter 10

1 Palmer, A. K. and Jensen, M. D. (2022). Metabolic changes in aging humans: current evidence and therapeutic strategies. *The Journal of Clinical Investigation*, *132*(16).
2 MacLean, P. S., Bergouignan, A., Cornier, M. A. and Jackman, M. R. (2011). Biology's response to dieting: the impetus for weight regain.

American Journal of Physiology-Regulatory, Integrative and Comparative Physiology, *301*(3), R581–600.
3   Blomain, E. S., Dirhan, D. A., Valentino, M. A., Kim, G. W. and Waldman, S. A. (2013). Mechanisms of weight regain following weight loss. *International Scholarly Research Notices*, *2013*(1), 210524.
4   Rand, K., Vallis, M., Aston, M., Price, S., Piccinini-Vallis, H., Rehman, L. and Kirk, S. F. (2017). 'It is not the diet; it is the mental part we need help with': a multilevel analysis of psychological, emotional, and social well-being in obesity. *International Journal of Qualitative Studies on Health and Well-being*, *12*(1), 1306421.
5   Espinosa-Salas, S. and Gonzalez-Arias, M. (2023). Nutrition: micronutrient intake, imbalances, and interventions. In *StatPearls* [Internet]. StatPearls Publishing.
6   Ibid.
7   Manore, M. M. (2005). Exercise and the Institute of Medicine recommendations for nutrition. *Current Sports Medicine Reports*, 4(4), 193–8.
8   Espinosa-Salas, S. and Gonzalez-Arias, M. (2023). Nutrition: micronutrient intake, imbalances, and interventions. In *StatPearls* [Internet]. StatPearls Publishing.
9   Sims, S. T., Kerksick, C. M., Smith-Ryan, A. E., Janse de Jonge, X. A., Hirsch, K. R., Arent, S. M., ... and Antonio, J. (2023). International Society of Sports Nutrition position stand: nutritional concerns of the female athlete. *Journal of the International Society of Sports Nutrition*, *20*(1), 2204066.
10 Manore, M. M. (2005). Exercise and the Institute of Medicine recommendations for nutrition. *Current Sports Medicine Reports*, 4(4), 193–8.
11 Espinosa-Salas, S. and Gonzalez-Arias, M. (2023). Nutrition: micronutrient intake, imbalances, and interventions. In *StatPearls* [Internet]. StatPearls Publishing.
12 Manore, M. M. (2005). Exercise and the Institute of Medicine recommendations for nutrition. *Current Sports Medicine Reports*, 4(4), 193–8.
13 https://www.nutrition.org.uk/nutritional-information/protein/
14 https://www.health.harvard.edu/nutrition/when-it-comes-to-protein-how-much-is-too-much
15 Volek, J. S., Forsythe, C. E. and Kraemer, W. J. (2006). Nutritional aspects of women strength athletes. *British Journal of Sports Medicine*, *40*(9), 742–8.
16 Gregorio, L., Brindisi, J., Kleppinger, A., Sullivan, R., Mangano, K. M., Bihuniak, J. D., ... and Insogn, K. L. (2014). Adequate dietary protein is associated with better physical performance among post-menopausal women 60–90 years. *The Journal of Nutrition, Health and Aging*, *18*(2), 155–60.

17 https://www.health.harvard.edu/nutrition/high-protein-foods-the-best-protein-sources-to-include-in-a-healthy-diet
18 Martinez-Lacoba, R., Pardo-Garcia, I., Amo-Saus, E. and Escribano-Sotos, F. (2018). Mediterranean diet and health outcomes: a systematic meta-review. *European Journal of Public Health*, *28*(5), 955–61.
19 Onwuzo, C., Olukorode, J. O., Omokore, O. A., Odunaike, O. S., Omiko, R., Osaghae, O. W., ... and Kristilere, H. (2023). DASH diet: a review of its scientifically proven hypertension reduction and health benefits. *Cureus*, *15*(9).
20 Derbyshire, E. J. (2017). Flexitarian diets and health: a review of the evidence-based literature. *Frontiers in Nutrition*, *3*, 231850.
21 Jafari, R. S. and Behrouz, V. (2023). Nordic diet and its benefits in neurological function: a systematic review of observational and intervention studies. *Frontiers in Nutrition*, *10*, 1215358.
22 Mahase, E. (2019). Vegetarian and pescatarian diets are linked to lower risk of ischaemic heart disease, study finds. *British Medical Journal*, *366*, l5397.
23 Hargreaves, S. M., Raposo, A., Saraiva, A. and Zandonadi, R. P. (2021). Vegetarian diet: an overview through the perspective of quality of life domains. *International Journal of Environmental Research and Public Health*, *18*(8), 4067.
24 Malhotra, A. and Lakade, A. (2025). Analytical review on nutritional deficiencies in vegan diets: risks, prevention, and optimal strategies. *Journal of the American Nutrition Association*, 1–11.
25 Masood, W., Annamaraju, P., Suheb, M. Z. K. and Uppaluri, K. R. (2023). Ketogenic diet. In *StatPearls* [Internet]. StatPearls Publishing.
26 Goedeke, S., Murphy, T., Rush, A. and Zinn, C. (2024). Assessing the nutrient composition of a carnivore diet: a case study model. *Nutrients*, *17*(1), 140.
27 Hartmann-Boyce, J., Theodoulou, A., Oke, J. L., Butler, A. R., Scarborough, P., Bastounis, A., ... and Aveyard, P. (2021). Association between characteristics of behavioural weight loss programmes and weight change after programme end: systematic review and meta-analysis. *British Medical Journal*, *374*.
28 Bóna, E., Forgács, A. and Túry, F. (2018). Potential relationship between juice cleanse diets and eating disorders: a qualitative pilot study. *Orvosi Hetilap*, *159*(28), 1153–7.
29 Most, J. and Redman, L. M. (2020). Impact of calorie restriction on energy metabolism in humans. *Experimental Gerontology*, *133*, 110875.
30 https://www.bhf.org.uk/informationsupport/heart-matters-magazine/nutrition/weight/diets/extreme-diets

31 Vetrani, C., Barrea, L., Rispoli, R., Verde, L., De Alteriis, G., Docimo, A., ... and Muscogiuri, G. (2022). Mediterranean diet: what are the consequences for menopause? *Frontiers in Endocrinology, 13*, 886824.
32 Gonçalves, C., Moreira, H. and Santos, R. (2024). Systematic review of Mediterranean diet interventions in menopausal women. *AIMS Public Health, 11*(1), 110.
33 Guasch-Ferré, M. and Willett, W. C. (2021). The Mediterranean diet and health: a comprehensive overview. *Journal of Internal Medicine, 290*(3), 549–66.
34 Widmer, R. J., Flammer, A. J., Lerman, L. O. and Lerman, A. (2015). The Mediterranean diet, its components, and cardiovascular disease. *The American Journal of Medicine, 128*(3), 229–38.
35 Boskou, D., Blekas, G. and Tsimidou, M. (2006). Olive oil composition. In *Olive Oil*, 2nd edn, ed. D. Boscou. Academic Press and AOCS Press. 1–72.
36 Schwingshackl, L., Christoph, M. and Hoffmann, G. (2015). Effects of olive oil on markers of inflammation and endothelial function: a systematic review and meta-analysis. *Nutrients, 7*(9), 7651–75.
37 Ussia, S., Ritorto, G., Mollace, R., Serra, M., Tavernese, A., Altomare, C., ... and Macrì, R. (2025). Exploring the benefits of extra virgin olive oil on cardiovascular health enhancement and disease prevention: a systematic review. *Nutrients, 17*(11), 1843.
38 Gonçalves, M., Vale, N. and Silva, P. (2024). Neuroprotective effects of olive oil: a comprehensive review of antioxidant properties. *Antioxidants, 13*(7), 762.
39 Markellos, C., Ourailidou, M. E., Gavriatopoulou, M., Halvatsiotis, P., Sergentanis, T. N. and Psaltopoulou, T. (2022). Olive oil intake and cancer risk: a systematic review and meta-analysis. *PLOS One, 17*(1), e0261649.
40 Fazlollahi, A., Motlagh Asghari, K., Aslan, C., Noori, M., Nejadghaderi, S. A., Araj-Khodaei, M., ... and Safiri, S. (2023). The effects of olive oil consumption on cognitive performance: a systematic review. *Frontiers in Nutrition, 10*, 1218538.
41 Denby, N. and Hobbs, S. (2011). *Nutrition for Dummies*, 2nd edn. For Dummies.
42 Lambert, R. (2024). *The Unprocessed Plate: Flavourful, UPF-free recipes to transform your health*. Dorling Kindersley.
43 https://www.nhlbi.nih.gov/health/overweight-and-obesity/causes
44 Razzoli, M., Pearson, C., Crow, S. and Bartolomucci, A. (2017). Stress, overeating, and obesity: insights from human studies and preclinical models. *Neuroscience & Biobehavioral Reviews, 76*, 154–62.

45 Rolls, B. J., Roe, L. S. and Meengs, J. S. (2006). Reductions in portion size and energy density of foods are additive and lead to sustained decreases in energy intake. *The American Journal of Clinical Nutrition*, *83*(1), 11–17.

46 Vargas-Alvarez, M. A., Navas-Carretero, S., Palla, L., Martínez, J. A. and Almiron-Roig, E. (2021). Impact of portion control tools on portion size awareness, choice and intake: systematic review and meta-analysis. *Nutrients*, *13*(6), 1978.

47 Garg, D., Smith, E. and Attuquayefio, T. (2025). Watching television while eating increases food intake: a systematic review and meta-analysis of experimental studies. *Nutrients*, *17*(1), 166.

48 Dritschel, B., Cooper, P. J. and Charnock, D. (1993). A problematic counter-regulation experiment: implications for the link between dietary restraint and overeating. *International Journal of Eating Disorders*, *13*(3), 297–304.

49 Zeballos, E. and Todd, J. E. (2020). The effects of skipping a meal on daily energy intake and diet quality. *Public Health Nutrition*, *23*(18), 3346–55; Ma, X., Chen, Q., Pu, Y., Guo, M., Jiang, Z., Huang, W., ... and Xu, Y. (2020). Skipping breakfast is associated with overweight and obesity: a systematic review and meta-analysis. *Obesity Research & Clinical Practice*, *14*(1), 1–8.

50 Basturk, B., Ozerson, Z. K. and Yuksel, A. (2021). Evaluation of the effect of macronutrients combination on blood sugar levels in healthy individuals. *Iranian Journal of Public Health*, *50*(2), 280.

51 Akhlaghi, M., Ghobadi, S., Zare, M. and Foshati, S. (2020). Effect of nuts on energy intake, hunger, and fullness, a systematic review and meta-analysis of randomized clinical trials. *Critical Reviews in Food Science and Nutrition*, *60*(1), 84–93.

52 Polivy, J., Herman, C. P. and Deo, R. (2010). Getting a bigger slice of the pie. Effects on eating and emotion in restrained and unrestrained eaters. *Appetite*, *55*(3), 426–30.

53 Torske, A., Bremer, B., Hölzel, B. K., Maczka, A. and Koch, K. (2024). Mindfulness meditation modulates stress-eating and its neural correlates. *Scientific Reports*, *14*(1), 7294.

54 Ledochowski, L., Ruedl, G., Taylor, A. H. and Kopp, M. (2015). Acute effects of brisk walking on sugary snack cravings in overweight people, affect and responses to a manipulated stress situation and to a sugary snack cue: a crossover study. *PlOS One*, *10*(3), e0119278.

55 Appelhans, B. M., Bleil, M. E., Waring, M. E., Schneider, K. L., Nackers, L. M., Busch, A. M., ... and Pagoto, S. L. (2013). Beverages contribute extra calories to meals and daily energy intake in overweight and obese women. *Physiology & Behavior*, *122*, 129–33; Chen, L., Appel, L. J., Loria, C., Lin, P. H., Champagne, C. M., Elmer, P. J., ... and Caballero,

B. (2009). Reduction in consumption of sugar-sweetened beverages is associated with weight loss: the PREMIER trial. *The American Journal of Clinical Nutrition*, *89*(5), 1299–306.
56. de Graaf, C. (2011). Why liquid energy results in overconsumption. *Proceedings of the Nutrition Society*, *70*(2), 162–70.
57. Schulze, M. B., Manson, J. E., Ludwig, D. S., Colditz, G. A., Stampfer, M. J., Willett, W. C. and Hu, F. B. (2004). Sugar-sweetened beverages, weight gain, and incidence of type-2 diabetes in young and middle-aged women. *Jama*, *292*(8), 927–34.
58. Takahashi, A. (2025). Can carbonated water support weight loss? *BMJ Nutrition, Prevention & Health*, *8*(1).
59. Carter, B. E. and Drewnowski, A. (2012). Beverages containing soluble fiber, caffeine, and green tea catechins suppress hunger and lead to less energy consumption at the next meal. *Appetite*, *59*(3), 755–61.
60. Sirotkin, A. V. and Kolesarova, A. (2021). The anti-obesity and health-promoting effects of tea and coffee. *Physiological Research*, *70*(2), 161.
61. Ha, O. R. and Lim, S. L. (2023). The role of emotion in eating behavior and decisions. *Frontiers in Psychology*, *14*, 1265074.
62. Barbee, K. G. and Timmerman, G. M. (2015). Emotional eating, nonpurge binge eating, and self-efficacy in healthy perimenopausal women. *Journal of Holistic Nursing*, *33*(4), 298–307; Anaya, C., Culbert, K. M. and Klump, K. L. (2023). Binge eating risk during midlife and the menopausal transition: sensitivity to ovarian hormones as potential mechanisms of risk. *Current Psychiatry Reports*, *25*(2), 45–52.
63. Costa, M. L., Costa, M. G. O., de Souza, M. F. C., da Silva, D. G., Vieira, D. A. D. S. and Mendes-Netto, R. S. (2021). Is physical activity protective against emotional eating associated factors during the COVID-19 pandemic? A cross-sectional study among physically active and inactive adults. *Nutrients*, *13*(11), 3861.
64. Frayn, M., Livshits, S. and Knäuper, B. (2018). Emotional eating and weight regulation: a qualitative study of compensatory behaviors and concerns. *Journal of Eating Disorders*, *6*, 1–10.
65. Vincent, C., Bodnaruc, A. M., Prud'homme, D., Guenette, J. and Giroux, I. (2024). Disordered eating behaviours during the menopausal transition: a systematic review. *Applied Physiology, Nutrition, and Metabolism*, *49*(10), 1286–308.
66. Yau, Y. H. and Potenza, M. N. (2013). Stress and eating behaviors. *Minerva Endocrinologica*, *38*(3), 255.
67. Wouters, S., Thewissen, V., Duif, M., van Bree, R. J., Lechner, L. and Jacobs, N. (2018). Habit strength and between-meal snacking in daily life: the moderating role of level of education. *Public Health Nutrition*, *21*(14), 2595–605.

68 Karine, D., Denis, P. H., Rémi, R. L., Irene, S., Martin, B., Jean-Marc, L. and Éric, D. (2013). Effects of the menopausal transition on dietary intake and appetite: a MONET Group study. *European Journal of Clinical Nutrition, 68*(2), 271.

69 Wu, T., Hou, X., Zhang, F., Sharma, M., Zhao, Y. and Shi, Z. (2020). Association between self-reported food preferences and psychological well-being during perimenopausal period among Chinese women. *Frontiers in Psychology, 11*, 1196.

70 https://www.mpg.de/24427625/0331-psy-what-drives-our-cravings-for-food-and-drink-155111

71 Corney, R. A., Sunderland, C. and James, L. J. (2016). Immediate pre-meal water ingestion decreases voluntary food intake in lean young males. *European Journal of Nutrition, 55*, 815–19.

72 Paddon-Jones, D., Westman, E., Mattes, R. D., Wolfe, R. R., Astrup, A. and Westerterp-Plantenga, M. (2008). Protein, weight management, and satiety. *The American Journal of Clinical Nutrition, 87*(5), 1558S–61S.

73 Wu, S., Jia, W., He, H., Yin, J., Xu, H., He, C., … and Cheng, R. (2023). A new dietary fiber can enhance satiety and reduce postprandial blood glucose in healthy adults: a randomized cross-over trial. *Nutrients, 15*(21), 4569.

74 Pereira, M. A., Erickson, E., McKee, P., Schrankler, K., Raatz, S. K., Lytle, L. A. and Pellegrini, A. D. (2011). Breakfast frequency and quality may affect glycemia and appetite in adults and children. *The Journal of Nutrition, 141*(1), 163–8.

75 Zeballos, E. and Todd, J. E. (2020). The effects of skipping a meal on daily energy intake and diet quality. *Public Health Nutrition, 23*(18), 3346–55.

76 Leidy, H. J., Tang, M., Armstrong, C. L., Martin, C. B. and Campbell, W. W. (2011). The effects of consuming frequent, higher-protein meals on appetite and satiety during weight loss in overweight/obese men. *Obesity, 19*(4), 818–24.

77 Nguyen, V., Cooper, L., Lowndes, J., Melanson, K., Angelopoulos, T. J., Rippe, J. M. and Reimers, K. (2012). Popcorn is more satiating than potato chips in normal-weight adults. *Nutrition Journal, 11*, 1–6.

78 Katz, D. L., Doughty, K. and Ali, A. (2011). Cocoa and chocolate in human health and disease. *Antioxidants & Redox Signaling, 15*(10), 2779–811.

79 Harshendra, G. and Reddy, K. R. (2023). Health benefits of yogurt – an ideal probiotic: a review. *International Journal of Science and Research, 12*(6), 2911–13.

80 Martin, L., Pahl, S., White, M. P. and May, J. (2019). Natural environments and craving: the mediating role of negative affect. *Health & Place, 58*, 102160.

81 Hagerman, C. J., Stock, M. L., Beekman, J. B., Yeung, E. W. and Persky, S. (2021). The ironic effects of dietary restraint in situations that undermine self-regulation. *Eating Behaviors*, 43, 101579.
82 Meier, B. P., Romano, A., Kateman, S. and Nori, R. (2023). Less is more: mindfulness, portion size, and candy eating pleasure. *Food Quality and Preference*, *103*, 104703.
83 Otterbring, T., Folwarczny, M. and Gasiorowska, A. (2024). The impact of hunger on indulgent food choices is moderated by healthy eating concerns. *Frontiers in Nutrition*, *11*, 1377120.
84 Bryazka, D., Reitsma, M. B., Griswold, M. G., Abate, K. H., Abbafati, C., Abbasi-Kangevari, M., ... and Diress, M. (2022). Population-level risks of alcohol consumption by amount, geography, age, sex, and year: a systematic analysis for the Global Burden of Disease Study 2020. *The Lancet*, *400*(10347), 185–235.
85 https://www.iarc.who.int/infographics/alcohol-and-cancer-in-the-who-european-region
86 Rehm, J., Samokhvalov, A. V. and Shield, K. D. (2013). Global burden of alcoholic liver diseases. *Journal of Hepatology*, *59*(1), 160–8.
87 https://world-heart-federation.org/news/no-amount-of-alcohol-is-good-for-the-heart-says-world-heart-federation/
88 Topiwala, A., Wang, C., Ebmeier, K. P., Burgess, S., Bell, S., Levey, D. F., ... and Nichols, T. E. (2022). Associations between moderate alcohol consumption, brain iron, and cognition in UK Biobank participants: observational and Mendelian randomization analyses. *PLoS Medicine*, *19*(7), e1004039.
89 Topiwala, A., Wang, C., Ebmeier, K. P., Burgess, S., Bell, S., Levey, D. F., ... and Nichols, T. E. (2022). Associations between moderate alcohol consumption, brain iron, and cognition in UK Biobank participants: observational and Mendelian randomization analyses. *PLoS Medicine*, *19*(7), e1004039.
90 Godos, J., Giampieri, F., Chisari, E., Micek, A., Paladino, N., Forbes-Hernández, T. Y., ... and Grosso, G. (2022). Alcohol consumption, bone mineral density, and risk of osteoporotic fractures: a dose–response meta-analysis. *International Journal of Environmental Research and Public Health*, *19*(3), 1515.
91 https://www.acc.org/About-ACC/Press-Releases/2024/03/28/11/58/alcohol-raises-heart-disease-risk-particularly-among-women
92 Colrain, I. M., Nicholas, C. L. and Baker, F. C. (2014). Alcohol and the sleeping brain. *Handbook of Clinical Neurology*, *125*, 415–31.
93 Yang, P. L., Heitkemper, M. M. and Kamp, K. J. (2021). Irritable bowel syndrome in midlife women: a narrative review. *Women's Midlife Health*, *7*(1), 4.

94 Heitkemper, M. M. and Chang, L. (2009). Do fluctuations in ovarian hormones affect gastrointestinal symptoms in women with irritable bowel syndrome? *Gender Medicine*, 6, 152–67.
95 Chen, C., Gong, X., Yang, X., Shang, X., Du, Q., Liao, Q., ... and Xu, J. (2019). The roles of estrogen and estrogen receptors in gastrointestinal disease. *Oncology Letters*, 18(6), 5673–80.
96 Cherpak, C. E. (2019). Mindful eating: a review of how the stress-digestion-mindfulness triad may modulate and improve gastrointestinal and digestive function. *Integrative Medicine: A Clinician's Journal*, 18(4), 48.
97 Baker, J. M., Al-Nakkash, L. and Herbst-Kralovetz, M. M. (2017). Estrogen–gut microbiome axis: physiological and clinical implications. *Maturitas*, 103, 45–53.
98 Liaquat, M., Minihane, A. M., Vauzour, D. and Pontifex, M. G. (2025). The gut microbiota in menopause: is there a role for prebiotic and probiotic solutions? *Post Reproductive Health*, 20533691251340491.
99 Mayer, E. (2016). *The Mind–Gut Connection: How the hidden conversation within our bodies impacts our mood, our choices, and our overall health.* Harper Wave.
100 https://www.grandviewresearch.com/industry-analysis/dietary-supplements-market-report
101 Ibid.
102 Lopresti, A. L., Smith, S. J., Malvi, H. and Kodgule, R. (2019). An investigation into the stress-relieving and pharmacological actions of an ashwagandha (*Withania somnifera*) extract: a randomized, double-blind, placebo-controlled study. *Medicine*, 98(37), e17186.
103 Leonard, M., Dickerson, B., Estes, L., Gonzalez, D. E., Jenkins, V., Johnson, S., ... and Kreider, R. B. (2024). Acute and repeated ashwagandha supplementation improves markers of cognitive function and mood. *Nutrients*, 16(12), 1813.
104 https://ods.od.nih.gov/factsheets/Ashwagandha-HealthProfessional/
105 Guo, S. and Rezaei, M. J. (2024). The benefits of ashwagandha (Withania somnifera) supplements on brain function and sports performance. *Frontiers in Nutrition*, 11, 1439294.
106 https://medlineplus.gov/druginfo/natural/953.html
107 Lima, G. A. C., Lima, P. D. A., Barros, M. D. G. C. R. M. D., Vardiero, L. P., Melo, E. F. D., Paranhos-Neto, F. D. P., ... and Farias, M. L. F. D. (2016). Calcium intake: good for the bones but bad for the heart? An analysis of clinical studies. *Archives of Endocrinology and Metabolism*, 60(3), 252–63.
108 Anderson, J. J., Kruszka, B., Delaney, J. A., He, K., Burke, G. L., Alonso, A., ... and Michos, E. D. (2016). Calcium intake from diet

and supplements and the risk of coronary artery calcification and its progression among older adults: 10-year follow-up of the Multi-Ethnic Study of Atherosclerosis (MESA). *Journal of the American Heart Association*, 5(10), e003815; Li, K., Wang, X. F., Li, D. Y., Chen, Y. C., Zhao, L. J., Liu, X. G., ... and Deng, H. W. (2018). The good, the bad, and the ugly of calcium supplementation: a review of calcium intake on human health. *Clinical Interventions in Aging*, 2443–52.

109 Smith-Ryan, A. E., Cabre, H. E., Eckerson, J. M. and Candow, D. G. (2021). Creatine supplementation in women's health: a lifespan perspective. *Nutrients*, 13(3), 877.

110 Kreider, R. B., Kalman, D. S., Antonio, J., Ziegenfuss, T. N., Wildman, R., Collins, R., ... and Lopez, H. L. (2017). International Society of Sports Nutrition position stand: safety and efficacy of creatine supplementation in exercise, sport, and medicine. *Journal of the International Society of Sports Nutrition*, 14(1), 18.

111 Marber, I. (2019). *ManFood: The no-nonsense guide to improving your health and energy in your 40s and beyond.* Piatkus.

112 Smith-Ryan, A. E., Cabre, H. E., Eckerson, J. M. and Candow, D. G. (2021). Creatine supplementation in women's health: a lifespan perspective. *Nutrients*, 13(3), 877.

113 Kaviani, M., Shaw, K. and Chilibeck, P. D. (2020). Benefits of creatine supplementation for vegetarians compared to omnivorous athletes: a systematic review. *International Journal of Environmental Research and Public Health*, 17(9), 3041.

114 Gualano, B., Macedo, A. R., Alves, C. R. R., Roschel, H., Benatti, F. B., Takayama, L., ... and Pereira, R. M. R. (2014). Creatine supplementation and resistance training in vulnerable older women: a randomized double-blind placebo-controlled clinical trial. *Experimental Gerontology*, 53, 7–15.

115 Ibid.

116 Xu, C., Bi, S., Zhang, W. and Luo, L. (2024). The effects of creatine supplementation on cognitive function in adults: a systematic review and meta-analysis. *Frontiers in Nutrition*, 11, 1424972.

117 Yokota, Y., Yamada, S., Yamamoto, D., Kato, K., Morito, A. and Takaoka, A. (2023). Creatine supplementation alleviates fatigue after exercise through anti-inflammatory action in skeletal muscle and brain. *Nutraceuticals*, 3(2), 234–49.

118 Chilibeck, P. D., Candow, D. G., Landeryou, T., Kaviani, M. and Paus-Jenssen, L. (2015). Effects of creatine and resistance training on bone health in postmenopausal women. *Medicine & Science in Sports & Exercise*, 47(8), 1587–95.

119 Doma, K., Ramachandran, A. K., Boullosa, D. and Connor, J. (2022). The paradoxical effect of creatine monohydrate on muscle damage markers: a systematic review and meta-analysis. *Sports Medicine*, 52(7), 1623–45.

120 Candow, D. G., Forbes, S. C., Roberts, M. D., Roy, B. D., Antonio, J., Smith-Ryan, A. E., ... and Roschel, H. (2022). Creatine o'clock: does timing of ingestion really influence muscle mass and performance? *Frontiers in Sports and Active Living*, 4, 893714.

121 Dinan, N. E., Hagele, A. M., Jagim, A. R., Miller, M. G. and Kerksick, C. M. (2022). Effects of creatine monohydrate timing on resistance training adaptations and body composition after 8 weeks in male and female collegiate athletes. *Frontiers in Sports and Active Living*, 4, 1033842.

122 Powers, M. E., Arnold, B. L., Weltman, A. L., Perrin, D. H., Mistry, D., Kahler, D. M., ... and Volek, J. (2003). Creatine supplementation increases total body water without altering fluid distribution. *Journal of Athletic Training*, 38(1), 44.

123 Rawson, E. S. (2018). The safety and efficacy of creatine monohydrate supplementation: what we have learned from the past 25 years of research. *Gatorade Sports Science Exchange*, 29, 1–6.

124 Antonio, J., Candow, D. G., Forbes, S. C., Gualano, B., Jagim, A. R., Kreider, R. B., ... and Ziegenfuss, T. N. (2021). Common questions and misconceptions about creatine supplementation: what does the scientific evidence really show? *Journal of the International Society of Sports Nutrition*, 18, 1–17.

125 Hosseini, H., Ghavidel, F., Rajabian, A., Homayouni-Tabrizi, M., Majeed, M. and Sahebkar, A. (2024). The effects of curcumin plus piperine co-administration on inflammation and oxidative stress: a systematic review and meta-analysis of randomized controlled trials. *Current Medicinal Chemistry*, 13(7), e70588.

126 Gupta, S. C., Patchva, S. and Aggarwal, B. B. (2013). Therapeutic roles of curcumin: lessons learned from clinical trials. *The AAPS Journal*, 15, 195–218.

127 Lopresti, A. L. (2018). The problem of curcumin and its bioavailability: could its gastrointestinal influence contribute to its overall health-enhancing effects? *Advances in Nutrition*, 9(1), 41–50.

128 Shoba, G., Joy, D., Joseph, T., Majeed, M., Rajendran, R. and Srinivas, P. S. S. R. (1998). Influence of piperine on the pharmacokinetics of curcumin in animals and human volunteers. *Planta Medica*, 64(4), 353–6.

129 https://ods.od.nih.gov/factsheets/VitaminD-HealthProfessional/

130 Holick, M. F. (2004). Sunlight and vitamin D for bone health and prevention of autoimmune diseases, cancers, and cardiovascular disease. *The American Journal of Clinical Nutrition*, 80(6), 1678S–88S.

131 Rebelos, E., Tentolouris, N. and Jude, E. (2023). The role of vitamin D in health and disease: a narrative review on the mechanisms linking vitamin D with disease and the effects of supplementation. *Drugs, 83*(8), 665–85.

132 Giustina, A., Bilezikian, J. P., Adler, R. A., Banfi, G., Bikle, D. D., Binkley, N. C., ... and Virtanen, J. K. (2024). Consensus statement on vitamin D status assessment and supplementation: whys, whens, and hows. *Endocrine Reviews, 45*(5), 625–54.

133 Fatima, G., Dzupina, A., Alhmadi, H. B., Magomedova, A., Siddiqui, Z., Mehdi, A., ... and MEHDI, A. (2024). Magnesium matters: a comprehensive review of its vital role in health and diseases. *Cureus, 16*(10).

134 Lindberg, J. S., Zobitz, M. M., Poindexter, J. R. and Pak, C. Y. (1990). Magnesium bioavailability from magnesium citrate and magnesium oxide. *Journal of the American College of Nutrition, 9*(1), 48–55.

135 Kapper, C., Oppelt, P., Ganhör, C., Gyunesh, A. A., Arbeithuber, B., Stelzl, P. and Rezk-Füreder, M. (2024). Minerals and the menstrual cycle: impacts on ovulation and endometrial health. *Nutrients, 16*(7), 1008.

136 Arab, A., Rafie, N., Amani, R. and Shirani, F. (2023). The role of magnesium in sleep health: a systematic review of available literature. *Biological Trace Element Research, 201*(1), 121–8; Mah, J. and Pitre, T. (2021). Oral magnesium supplementation for insomnia in older adults: a systematic review & meta-analysis. *BMC Complementary Medicine and Therapies, 21*, 1–11.

137 Park, H., Parker, G. L., Boardman, C. H., Morris, M. M. and Smith, T. J. (2011). A pilot phase II trial of magnesium supplements to reduce menopausal hot flashes in breast cancer patients. *Supportive Care in Cancer, 19*, 859–63.

138 Orchard, T. S., Larson, J. C., Alghothani, N., Bout-Tabaku, S., Cauley, J. A., Chen, Z., ... and Jackson, R. D. (2014). Magnesium intake, bone mineral density, and fractures: results from the Women's Health Initiative Observational Study. *The American Journal of Clinical Nutrition, 99*(4), 926–33.

139 Blancquaert, L., Vervaet, C. and Derave, W. (2019). Predicting and testing bioavailability of magnesium supplements. *Nutrients, 11*(7), 1663.

140 Costello, R., Rosanoff, A., Nielsen, F. and West, C. (2023). Perspective: call for re-evaluation of the tolerable upper intake level for magnesium supplementation in adults. *Advances in Nutrition, 14*(5), 973–82.

141 Antonio, J., Evans, C., Ferrando, A. A., Stout, J. R., Antonio, B., Cintineo, H. P., ... and Kreider, R. B. (2024). Common questions and misconceptions about protein supplementation: what does the scientific evidence really show? *Journal of the International Society of Sports Nutrition, 21*(1), 2341903.

142 Pudasainee, P. and Anjum, F. (2020). *Protein Intolerance*. StatPearls [Internet].
143 Langyan, S., Yadava, P., Khan, F. N., Dar, Z. A., Singh, R. and Kumar, A. (2022). Sustaining protein nutrition through plant-based foods. *Frontiers in Nutrition, 8*, 772573.
144 https://ods.od.nih.gov/factsheets/Omega3FattyAcids-HealthProfessional/
145 Kavyani, Z., Musazadeh, V., Fathi, S., Faghfouri, A. H., Dehghan, P. and Sarmadi, B. (2022). Efficacy of the omega-3 fatty acids supplementation on inflammatory biomarkers: an umbrella meta-analysis. *International Immunopharmacology, 111*, 109104.
146 Wang, T., Zhang, X., Zhou, N., Shen, Y., Li, B., Chen, B. E. and Li, X. (2023). Association between omega-3 fatty acid intake and dyslipidemia: a continuous dose–response meta-analysis of randomized controlled trials. *Journal of the American Heart Association, 12*(11), e029512.
147 Khan, S. U., Lone, A. N., Khan, M. S., Virani, S. S., Blumenthal, R. S., Nasir, K., ... and Bhatt, D. L. (2021). Effect of omega-3 fatty acids on cardiovascular outcomes: a systematic review and meta-analysis. *eClinicalMedicine, 38*.
148 Dighriri, I. M., Alsubaie, A. M., Hakami, F. M., Hamithi, D. M., Alshekh, M. M., Khobrani, F. A., ... and Tawhari, M. (2022). Effects of omega-3 polyunsaturated fatty acids on brain functions: a systematic review. *Cureus, 14*(10).
149 Kuszewski, J. C., Wong, R. H. and Howe, P. R. (2020). Fish oil supplementation reduces osteoarthritis-specific pain in older adults with overweight/obesity. *Rheumatology Advances in Practice, 4*(2), rkaa036.
150 Tóth-Mészáros, A., Garmaa, G., Hegyi, P., Bánvölgyi, A., Fenyves, B., Fehérvári, P., ... and Csupor, D. (2023). The effect of adaptogenic plants on stress: a systematic review and meta-analysis. *Journal of Functional Foods, 108*, 105695.
151 Tinsley, G. M., Jagim, A. R., Potter, G. D., Garner, D. and Galpin, A. J. (2024). *Rhodiola rosea* as an adaptogen to enhance exercise performance: a review of the literature. *British Journal of Nutrition, 131*(3), 461–73.
152 Ross, S. M. (2023). The clinical efficacy of *Rhodiola rosea* L. in managing stress-induced conditions. *Holistic Nursing Practice, 37*(4), 233–5.
153 Spasov, A. A., Wikman, G. K., Mandrikov, V. B., Mironova, I. A. and Neumoin, V. V. (2000). A double-blind, placebo-controlled pilot study of the stimulating and adaptogenic effect of *Rhodiola rosea* SHR-5 extract on the fatigue of students caused by stress during an examination period with a repeated low-dose regimen. *Phytomedicine, 7*(2), 85–9.

Chapter 11

1. Xu, H., Liu, J., Li, P. and Liang, Y. (2024). Effects of mind–body exercise on perimenopausal and postmenopausal women: a systematic review and meta-analysis. *Menopause, 31*(5), 457–67.
2. Lin, Z., Shi, G., Liao, X., Huang, J., Yu, M., Liu, W., ... and Cai, X. (2023). Correlation between sedentary activity, physical activity and bone mineral density and fat in America: National Health and Nutrition Examination Survey, 2011–18. *Scientific Reports, 13*(1), 10054; Warburton, D. E., Nicol, C. W. and Bredin, S. S. (2006). Health benefits of physical activity: the evidence. *Cmaj, 174*(6), 801–9.
3. Jayedi, A., Soltani, S., Motlagh, S. Z. T., Emadi, A., Shahinfar, H., Moosavi, H. and Shab-Bidar, S. (2022). Anthropometric and adiposity indicators and risk of type 2 diabetes: systematic review and dose–response meta-analysis of cohort studies. *British Medical Journal, 376*, e067516.
4. Samargandy, S., Matthews, K. A., Brooks, M. M., Barinas-Mitchell, E., Magnani, J. W., Janssen, I., ... and El Khoudary, S. R. (2021). Abdominal visceral adipose tissue over the menopause transition and carotid atherosclerosis: the SWAN heart study. *Menopause, 28*(6), 626–33.
5. Lauby-Secretan, B., Scoccianti, C., Loomis, D., Grosse, Y., Bianchini, F. and Straif, K. (2016). Body fatness and cancer: viewpoint of the IARC Working Group. *New England Journal of Medicine, 375*(8), 794–8.
6. Dąbrowska-Galas, M. and Dąbrowska, J. (2021). Physical activity level and self-esteem in middle-aged women. *International Journal of Environmental Research and Public Health, 18*(14), 7293.
7. https://www.gov.uk/government/publications/physical-activity-guidelines-uk-chief-medical-officers-report
8. https://www.sportengland.org/research-and-data/data/active-lives
9. Sport England (2025). Active Lives Adult Survey: November 2022 to November 2023 report. Available at: https://sportengland-production-files.s3.eu-west-2.amazonaws.com/s3fs-public/2025–04/ActiveLivesAdult-Nov23-24_V9-23-04-25-10-03-03-02.pdf
10. https://womeninsport.org/resource/menopause/
11. Capel-Alcaraz, A. M., García-López, H., Castro-Sánchez, A. M., Fernández-Sánchez, M. and Lara-Palomo, I. C. (2023). The efficacy of strength exercises for reducing the symptoms of menopause: a systematic review. *Journal of Clinical Medicine, 12*(2), 548.
12. Keawtep, P., Wichayanrat, W., Boripuntakul, S., Chattipakorn, S. C. and Sungkarat, S. (2022). Cognitive benefits of physical exercise, physical–cognitive training, and technology-based intervention in obese individuals with and without postmenopausal condition: a narrative review. *International Journal of Environmental Research and Public Health, 19*(20), 13364.

13 Xu, H., Liu, J., Li, P. and Liang, Y. (2024). Effects of mind–body exercise on perimenopausal and postmenopausal women: a systematic review and meta-analysis. *Menopause, 31*(5), 457–67.
14 Bailey, T. G., Cable, N. T., Aziz, N., Dobson, R., Sprung, V. S., Low, D. A. and Jones, H. (2016). Exercise training reduces the frequency of menopausal hot flushes by improving thermoregulatory control. *Menopause, 23*(7), 708–18.
15 Sternfeld, B. and Dugan, S. (2011). Physical activity and health during the menopausal transition. *Obstetrics and Gynecology Clinics of North America, 38*(3), 537.
16 Karacan, S. (2010). Effects of long-term aerobic exercise on physical fitness and postmenopausal symptoms with menopausal rating scale. *Science & Sports, 25*(1), 39–46.
17 Lee, D. C. and Schroeder, E. C. (2016). Resistance training improves cardiovascular health in postmenopausal women. *Menopause, 23*(11), 1162–4.
18 Bueno-Notivol, J., Calvo-Latorre, J., Alonso-Ventura, V., Pasupuleti, V., Hernandez, A. V. and Perez-Lopez, F. R. (2017). Effect of programmed exercise on insulin sensitivity in postmenopausal women: a systematic review and meta-analysis of randomized controlled trials. *Menopause, 24*(12), 1404–13.
19 Thomas, E., Gentile, A., Lakicevic, N., Moro, T., Bellafiore, M., Paoli, A., ... and Bianco, A. (2021). The effect of resistance training programs on lean body mass in postmenopausal and elderly women: a meta-analysis of observational studies. *Aging Clinical and Experimental Research, 33*(11), 2941–52.
20 Walsh, G. S., Delextrat, A. and Bibbey, A. (2023). The comparative effect of exercise interventions on balance in perimenopausal and early postmenopausal women: a systematic review and network meta-analysis of randomised, controlled trials. *Maturitas, 175*, 107790.
21 Wang, Z., Zan, X., Li, Y., Lu, Y., Xia, Y. and Pan, X. (2023). Comparative efficacy different resistance training protocols on bone mineral density in postmenopausal women: a systematic review and network meta-analysis. *Frontiers in Physiology, 14*, 1105303.
22 Keawtep, P., Sungkarat, S., Boripuntakul, S., Sa-Nguanmoo, P., Wichayanrat, W., Chattipakorn, S. C. and Worakul, P. (2024). Effects of combined dietary intervention and physical-cognitive exercise on cognitive function and cardiometabolic health of postmenopausal women with obesity: a randomized controlled trial. *International Journal of Behavioral Nutrition and Physical Activity, 21*(1), 28; Karamacoska, D., Butt, A., Leung, I. H., Childs, R. L., Metri, N. J., Uruthiran, V., ... and Steiner-Lim, G. Z. (2023). Brain

function effects of exercise interventions for cognitive decline: a systematic review and meta-analysis. *Frontiers in Neuroscience, 17*, 1127065.

23 Poon, E. T. C., Li, H. Y., Little, J. P., Wong, S. H. S. and Ho, R. S. T. (2024). Efficacy of interval training in improving body composition and adiposity in apparently healthy adults: an umbrella review with meta-analysis. *Sports Medicine, 54*(11), 2817–40.

24 Liu, C. J. and Latham, N. K. (2009). Progressive resistance strength training for improving physical function in older adults. *Cochrane Database of Systematic Reviews*, 3:CD002759.

25 Capel-Alcaraz, A. M., García-López, H., Castro-Sánchez, A. M., Fernández-Sánchez, M. and Lara-Palomo, I. C. (2023). The efficacy of strength exercises for reducing the symptoms of menopause: a systematic review. *Journal of Clinical Medicine, 12*(2), 548.

26 Marcos-Pardo, P. J., Vaquero-Cristóbal, R., and Huber, G. (2023). The power of resistance training: Evidence-based recommendations for middle-aged and older women's health. *Retos*, 51, 319–331.

27 Li, Y. and Fang, J. (2024). The impact of high-intensity interval training on women's health: a bibliometric and visualization analysis. *Medicine, 103*(39), e39855.

28 Vetrovsky, T., Steffl, M., Stastny, P. and Tufano, J. J. (2019). The efficacy and safety of lower-limb plyometric training in older adults: a systematic review. *Sports Medicine, 49*, 113–31; An, J., Su, Z. and Meng, S. (2024). Effect of aerobic training versus resistance training for improving cardiorespiratory fitness and body composition in middle-aged to older adults: a systematic review and meta-analysis of randomized controlled trials. *Archives of Gerontology and Geriatrics, 126*, 105530.

29 Lee, D., Son, J. Y., Ju, H. M., Won, J. H., Park, S. B. and Yang, W. H. (2021). Effects of individualized low-intensity exercise and its duration on recovery ability in adults. *Healthcare, 9*, 249.

30 An, J., Su, Z. and Meng, S. (2024). Effect of aerobic training versus resistance training for improving cardiorespiratory fitness and body composition in middle-aged to older adults: a systematic review and meta-analysis of randomized controlled trials. *Archives of Gerontology and Geriatrics, 126*, 105530.

31 Vasudevan, A. and Ford, E. (2022). Motivational factors and barriers towards initiating and maintaining strength training in women: a systematic review and meta-synthesis. *Prevention Science, 23*(4), 674–95.

32 Peng, B., Ng, J. Y. and Ha, A. S. (2023). Barriers and facilitators to physical activity for young adult women: a systematic review and thematic synthesis of qualitative literature. *International Journal of Behavioral Nutrition and Physical Activity, 20*(1), 23.

33 Sims, S. T., Kerksick, C. M., Smith-Ryan, A. E., Janse de Jonge, X. A., Hirsch, K. R., Arent, S. M., ... and Antonio, J. (2023). International Society of Sports Nutrition position stand: nutritional concerns of the female athlete. *Journal of the International Society of Sports Nutrition*, *20*(1), 2204066.

34 Vardardottir, B., Gudmundsdottir, S. L., Tryggvadottir, E. A. and Olafsdottir, A. S. (2024). Patterns of energy availability and carbohydrate intake differentiate between adaptable and problematic low energy availability in female athletes. *Frontiers in Sports and Active Living*, *6*, 1390558.

35 Hoyenga, K. B. and Hoyenga, K. T. (1982). Gender and energy balance: sex differences in adaptations for feast and famine. *Physiology & Behavior*, *28*(3), 545–63.

36 Greenleaf, C. and Hauff, C. (2024). 'When it fits wrong, I'm so self-conscious I want to die!': women's experiences wearing plus-size exercise clothing. *Sex Roles*, *90*(10), 1381–92.

37 Geraci, A., Calvani, R., Ferri, E., Marzetti, E., Arosio, B. and Cesari, M. (2021). Sarcopenia and menopause: the role of estradiol. *Frontiers in Endocrinology*, *12*, 682012.

38 Zhang, C., Feng, X., Zhang, X., Chen, Y., Kong, J. and Lou, Y. (2024). Research progress on the correlation between estrogen and estrogen receptor on postmenopausal sarcopenia. *Frontiers in Endocrinology*, *15*, 1494972.

39 Buckinx, F. and Aubertin-Leheudre, M. (2022). Sarcopenia in menopausal women: current perspectives. *International Journal of Women's Health*, 805–19.

40 https://theros.org.uk/about-us/media-centre/media-toolkit

41 Ji, M. X. and Yu, Q. (2015). Primary osteoporosis in postmenopausal women. *Chronic Diseases and Translational Medicine*, *1*(01), 9–13.

42 Bone Health & Osteoporosis Foundation (BHOF) (n.d.). Osteoporosis: fast facts. Available at: https://www.bonehealthandosteoporosis.org/wp-content/uploads/Osteoporosis-Fast-Facts-2.pdf

43 Mohebbi, R., Shojaa, M., Kohl, M., von Stengel, S., Jakob, F., Kerschan-Schindl, K., ... and Kemmler, W. (2023). Exercise training and bone mineral density in postmenopausal women: an updated systematic review and meta-analysis of intervention studies with emphasis on potential moderators. *Osteoporosis International*, *34*(7), 1145–78; Rathleff, M. S., Mølgaard, C. M., Fredberg, U., Kaalund, S., Andersen, K. B., Jensen, T. T., ... and Olesen, J. L. (2015). High-load strength training improves outcome in patients with plantar fasciitis: a randomized controlled trial with 12-month follow-up. *Scandinavian Journal of Medicine & Science in Sports*, *25*(3), e292–e300.

44 Lee, J. H., Jeon, H. G. and Yoon, Y. J. (2023, May). Effects of exercise intervention (with and without joint mobilization) in patients with adhesive capsulitis: a systematic review and meta-analysis. *Healthcare, 11*(10), 504.
45 Kolnes, K. J., Petersen, M. H., Lien-Iversen, T., Højlund, K. and Jensen, J. (2021). Effect of exercise training on fat loss: energetic perspectives and the role of improved adipose tissue function and body fat distribution. *Frontiers in Physiology, 12*, 737709.
46 Poehlman, E. T., Dvorak, R. V., DeNino, W. F., Brochu, M. and Ades, P. A. (2000). Effects of resistance training and endurance training on insulin sensitivity in nonobese, young women: a controlled randomized trial. *The Journal of Clinical Endocrinology & Metabolism, 85*(7), 2463–8.
47 Greer, B. K., O'Brien, J. U. L. I. E., Hornbuckle, L. M. and Panton, L. B. (2021). EPOC comparison between resistance training and high-intensity interval training in aerobically fit women. *International Journal of Exercise Science, 14*(2), 1027.
48 Eidukaitė, S., Masiulis, N. and Kvedaras, M. (2023). Exploring the preliminary effects of resistance training on total brain-derived neurotrophic factor (BDNF) levels in elderly individuals: a pilot study. *Baltic Journal of Sport and Health Sciences, 2*(129), 4–10.
49 Liu-Ambrose, T., Nagamatsu, L. S., Graf, P., Beattie, B. L., Ashe, M. C. and Handy, T. C. (2010). Resistance training and executive functions: a 12-month randomized controlled trial. *Archives of Internal Medicine, 170*(2), 170–8; Broadhouse, K. M., Singh, M. F., Suo, C., Gates, N., Wen, W., Brodaty, H., ... and Valenzuela, M. J. (2020). Hippocampal plasticity underpins long-term cognitive gains from resistance exercise in MCI. *NeuroImage: Clinical, 25*, 102182.
50 Anderson, E. and Shivakumar, G. (2013). Effects of exercise and physical activity on anxiety. *Frontiers in Psychiatry, 4*, 27.
51 Wender, C. L., Manninen, M. and O'Connor, P. J. (2022). The effect of chronic exercise on energy and fatigue states: a systematic review and meta-analysis of randomized trials. *Frontiers in Psychology, 13*, 907637; Kovacevic, A., Mavros, Y., Heisz, J. J. and Singh, M. A. F. (2018). The effect of resistance exercise on sleep: a systematic review of randomized controlled trials. *Sleep Medicine Reviews, 39*, 52–68.
52 Streetman, A. E., Lister, M. M., Brown, A., Brin, H. N. and Heinrich, K. M. (2023). A mixed-methods study of women's empowerment through physical activities: relationships with self-efficacy and physical activity levels. *Journal of Functional Morphology and Kinesiology, 8*(3), 118.
53 Sims, S. and Yeager, C. (2023). *ROAR: Fitness, physiology & nutrition for optimising female performance*, rev. edn. Rodale Books.

54 Wu, Y., Wang, W., Liu, T. and Zhang, D. (2017). Association of grip strength with risk of all-cause mortality, cardiovascular diseases, and cancer in community-dwelling populations: a meta-analysis of prospective cohort studies. *Journal of the American Medical Directors Association*, *18*(6), 551-e17; Wang, Y., Luo, D., Liu, J., Song, Y., Jiang, B. and Jiang, H. (2023). Low skeletal muscle mass index and all-cause mortality risk in adults: a systematic review and meta-analysis of prospective cohort studies. *PLOS One*, *18*(6), e0286745; Kodama, S., Saito, K., Tanaka, S., Maki, M., Yachi, Y., Asumi, M., ... and Sone, H. (2009). Cardiorespiratory fitness as a quantitative predictor of all-cause mortality and cardiovascular events in healthy men and women: a meta-analysis. *Jama*, *301*(19), 2024–35.
55 Yang, X. P. and Reckelhoff, J. F. (2011). Estrogen, hormonal replacement therapy and cardiovascular disease. *Current Opinion in Nephrology and Hypertension*, *20*(2), 13–8.
56 British Heart Foundation (2025, January). Cardiovascular disease statistics: UK factsheet. https://www.bhf.org.uk/-/media/files/for-professionals/research/heart-statistics/bhf-cvd-statistics-uk-factsheet.pdf
57 Li, T. and Zhang, L. (2023). Effect of exercise on cardiovascular risk in sedentary postmenopausal women: a systematic review and meta-analysis. *Annals of Palliative Medicine*, *12*(1), 15062–162; Hulteen, R. M., Marlatt, K. L., Allerton, T. D. and Lovre, D. (2023). Detrimental changes in health during menopause: the role of physical activity. *International Journal of Sports Medicine*, *44*(06), 389–96.
58 Kodoth, V., Scaccia, S. and Aggarwal, B. (2022). Adverse changes in body composition during the menopausal transition and relation to cardiovascular risk: a contemporary review. *Women's Health Reports*, *3*(1), 573–81.
59 Vecchiatto, B., Castro, T. L., Ferreira, N. J. R. and Evangelista, F. S. (2025). Healthy adipose tissue after menopause: contribution of balanced diet and physical exercise. *Exploration of Endocrine and Metabolic Diseases*, *2*, 101424.
60 Hyvärinen, M., Juppi, H. K., Taskinen, S., Karppinen, J. E., Karvinen, S., Tammelin, T. H., ... and Laakkonen, E. K. (2022). Metabolic health, menopause, and physical activity: a 4-year follow-up study. *International Journal of Obesity*, *46*(3), 544–54; Ross, R., Janssen, I., Dawson, J., Kungl, A. M., Kuk, J. L., Wong, S. L., ... and Hudson, R. (2004). Exercise-induced reduction in obesity and insulin resistance in women: a randomized controlled trial. *Obesity Research*, *12*(5), 789–98.
61 Hunter, M. R., Gillespie, B. W. and Chen, S. Y. P. (2019). Urban nature experiences reduce stress in the context of daily life based on salivary biomarkers. *Frontiers in Psychology*, *10*, 413490.

62 Anderson, E. and Shivakumar, G. (2013). Effects of exercise and physical activity on anxiety. *Frontiers in Psychiatry*, *4*, 27; Alnawwar, M. A., Alraddadi, M. I., Algethmi, R. A., Salem, G. A., Salem, M. A. and Alharbi, A. A. (2023). The effect of physical activity on sleep quality and sleep disorder: a systematic review. *Cureus*, *15*(8).

63 Liu, K., Zhao, W., Li, C., Tian, Y., Wang, L., Zhong, J., ... and Wang, H. (2024). The effects of high-intensity interval training on cognitive performance: a systematic review and meta-analysis. *Scientific Reports*, *14*(1), 32082.

64 Stamatis, A., Morgan, G. B., Boolani, A. and Papadakis, Z. (2024). The positive association between grit and mental toughness, enhanced by a minimum of 75 minutes of moderate-to-vigorous physical activity, among US students. *Psych*, *6*(1), 221–35.

65 Wicks, C., Barton, J., Orbell, S. and Andrews, L. (2022). Psychological benefits of outdoor physical activity in natural versus urban environments: a systematic review and meta-analysis of experimental studies. *Applied Psychology: Health and Well-Being*, *14*(3), 1037–61.

66 Marselle, M. R., Irvine, K. N. and Warber, S. L. (2013). Walking for well-being: are group walks in certain types of natural environments better for well-being than group walks in urban environments? *International Journal of Environmental Research and Public Health*, *10*(11), 5603–28.

67 Barton, J. and Pretty, J. (2010). What is the best dose of nature and green exercise for improving mental health? A multi-study analysis. *Environmental Science & Technology*, *44*(10), 3947–55.

Chapter 12

1 Scavello, I., Maseroli, E., Di Stasi, V. and Vignozzi, L. (2019). Sexual health in menopause. *Medicina*, *55*(9), 559.

2 Kingsberg, S. A., Schaffir, J., Faught, B. M., Pinkerton, J. V., Parish, S. J., Iglesia, C. B., ... and Simon, J. A. (2019). Female sexual health: barriers to optimal outcomes and a roadmap for improved patient–clinician communications. *Journal of Women's Health*, *28*(4), 432–43.

3 https://www.swanstudy.org/

4 Avis, N. E., Zhao, X., Johannes, C. B., Ory, M., Brockwell, S. and Greendale, G. A. (2005). Correlates of sexual function among multi-ethnic middle-aged women: results from the Study of Women's Health Across the Nation (SWAN). *Menopause*, *12*(4), 385–98.

5 Waetjen, L. E., Johnson, W. O., Xing, G., Hess, R., Avis, N. E., Reed, B. D., ... and Study of Women's Health Across the Nation (SWAN) (2022). Patterns of sexual activity and the development of sexual pain across the menopausal transition. *Obstetrics & Gynecology*, *139*(6), 1130–40.

6. Waetjen, L. E., Crawford, S. L., Chang, P. Y., Reed, B. D., Hess, R., Avis, N. E., ... and Gold, E. B. (2018). Factors associated with developing vaginal dryness symptoms in women transitioning through menopause: a longitudinal study. *Menopause*, *25*(10), 1094–104.
7. Khani, S., Azizi, M., Elyasi, F., Kamali, M. and Moosazadeh, M. (2021). The prevalence of sexual dysfunction in the different menopausal stages: a systematic review and meta-analysis. *International Journal of Sexual Health*, *33*(3), 439–72.
8. Herkommer, K., Meissner, V. H., Dinkel, A., Jahnen, M., Schiele, S., Kron, M., ... and Gschwend, J. E. (2024). Prevalence, lifestyle, and risk factors of erectile dysfunction, premature ejaculation, and low libido in middle-aged men: first results of the Bavarian Men's Health-Study. *Andrology*, *12*(4), 801–8.
9. Mark, K. P., Arenella, K., Girard, A., Herbenick, D., Fu, J. and Coleman, E. (2024). Erectile dysfunction prevalence in the United States: report from the 2021 National Survey of Sexual Wellbeing. *The Journal of Sexual Medicine*, *21*(4), 296–303.
10. Maiorino, M. I., Bellastella, G. and Esposito, K. (2015). Lifestyle modifications and erectile dysfunction: what can be expected? *Asian Journal of Andrology*, *17*(1), 5–10.
11. Patoulias, D., Katsimardou, A., Imprialos, K. and Doumas, M. (2022). Exercise, erectile dysfunction and co-morbidities: 'the good, the bad and the ugly'. *Reviews in Cardiovascular Medicine*, *23*(9), 304.
12. Meldrum, D. R., Gambone, J. C., Morris, M. A., Meldrum, D. A., Esposito, K. and Ignarro, L. J. (2011). The link between erectile and cardiovascular health: the canary in the coal mine. *The American Journal of Cardiology*, *108*(4), 599–606.
13. https://www.gminsights.com/industry-analysis/erectile-dysfunction-drugs-market
14. Bhupathiraju, S. N., Grodstein, F., Stampfer, M. J., Willett, W. C., Crandall, C. J., Shifren, J. L. and Manson, J. E. (2019). Vaginal estrogen use and chronic disease risk in the Nurses' Health Study. *Menopause*, *26*(6), 603–10.
15. Dennerstein, L., Randolph, J., Taffe, J., Dudley, E. and Burger, H. (2002). Hormones, mood, sexuality, and the menopausal transition. *Fertility and Sterility*, *77*, 42–8.
16. Kasano, J. P. M., Crespo, H. F. G., Arias, R. A. R. and Alamo, I. (2023). Genitourinary syndrome in menopause: impact of vaginal symptoms. *Turkish Journal of Obstetrics and Gynecology*, *20*(1), 38.
17. Edwards, D. and Panay, N. (2016). Treating vulvovaginal atrophy/genitourinary syndrome of menopause: how important is vaginal lubricant and moisturizer composition? *Climacteric*, *19*(2), 151–61.

18 Antônio, F. I., Herbert, R. D., Bø, K., Rosa-e, A. C. J. S., Lara, L. A. S., de Menezes Franco, M. and Ferreira, C. H. J. (2018). Pelvic floor muscle training increases pelvic floor muscle strength more in post-menopausal women who are not using hormone therapy than in women who are using hormone therapy: a randomised trial. *Journal of Physiotherapy*, *64*(3), 166–71; Zhuo, Z., Wang, C., Yu, H. and Li, J. (2021). The relationship between pelvic floor function and sexual function in perimenopausal women. *Sexual Medicine*, *9*(6), 100441.

19 Jokar, F., Fani, M., Isfahani, N. T. and Sabahi, R. (2025). Effectiveness of biofeedback with dilator therapy for sexual function in women with primary vaginismus: randomized controlled trial study. *International Urogynecology Journal*, *36*(3), 557–65.

20 Lara, L. A., Cartagena-Ramos, D., Figueiredo, J. B., Rosa-e-Silva, A. C. J., Ferriani, R. A., Martins, W. P. and Fuentealba-Torres, M. (2023). Hormone therapy for sexual function in perimenopausal and postmenopausal women. *Cochrane Database of Systematic Reviews* (8).

21 Rahn, D. D., Carberry, C., Sanses, T. V., Mamik, M. M., Ward, R. M., Meriwether, K. V., ... and Society of Gynecologic Surgeons Systematic Review Group. (2014). Vaginal estrogen for genitourinary syndrome of menopause: a systematic review. *Obstetrics & Gynecology*, *124*(6), 1147–56.

22 https://www.nia.nih.gov/health/menopause/sex-and-menopause-treatment-symptoms

23 Fang, Y., Liu, F., Zhang, X., Chen, L., Liu, Y., Yang, L., ... and Li, Z. (2024). Mapping global prevalence of menopausal symptoms among middle-aged women: a systematic review and meta-analysis. *BMC Public Health*, *24*(1), 1767.

24 Jaderek, I. and Lew-Starowicz, M. (2019). A systematic review on mindfulness meditation-based interventions for sexual dysfunctions. *The Journal of Sexual Medicine*, *16*(10), 1581–96.

25 Khaddouma, A., Coop Gordon, K. and Strand, E. B. (2017). Mindful mates: pilot study of the relational effects of mindfulness-based stress reduction on participants and their partners. *Family Process*, *56*(3), 636–51.

26 https://news.iu.edu/live/news/44923-kinsey-institute-releases-new-research-revealing-major

27 Kılıç, D., Armstrong, H. L. and Graham, C. A. (2023). The role of mutual masturbation within relationships: associations with sexual satisfaction and sexual self-esteem. *International Journal of Sexual Health*, *35*(4), 495–514.

28 Kuck, M. J. and Hogervorst, E. (2024). Stress, depression, and anxiety: psychological complaints across menopausal stages. *Frontiers in Psychiatry*, *15*, 1323743; Refaei, M., Mardanpour, S., Masoumi, S. Z. and Parsa, P. (2022). Women's experiences in the transition to menopause:

a qualitative research. *BMC Women's Health*, *22*(1), 53; Anto, A., Basu, A., Selim, R. and Eisingerich, A. B. (2025). Women's menopausal experiences in the UK: a systemic literature review of qualitative studies. *Health Expectations*, *28*(1), e70167.

29 Mark, K. P., Vowels, L. M., Mullis, L. and Hoskins, K. (2023). Women's strategies for navigating a healthy sex life post-sexual trauma. *PlOS One*, *18*(9), e0291011.

30 Van Lankveld, J., Jacobs, N., Thewissen, V., Dewitte, M. and Verboon, P. (2018). The associations of intimacy and sexuality in daily life: temporal dynamics and gender effects within romantic relationships. *Journal of Social and Personal relationships*, *35*(4), 557–76.

31 Kling, J. M., Kapoor, E., Mara, K. and Faubion, S. S. (2021). Associations of sleep and female sexual function: good sleep quality matters. *Menopause*, *28*(6), 619–25; Heidari, M., Ghodusi, M., Rezaei, P., Abyaneh, S. K., Sureshjani, E. H. and Sheikhi, R. A. (2019). Sexual function and factors affecting menopause: a systematic review. *Journal of Menopausal Medicine*, *25*(1), 15–27.

32 Fraser, A. M., Leavitt, C. E., Yorgason, J. B. and Price, A. A. (2023). 'Feeling it': links between elements of compassion and sexual well-being. *Frontiers in Psychology*, *13*, 1017384.

33 de Boer, M. (2025). 'Becumming' oneself as one relates to others: an empirical phenomenological study about sexual identity work in menopause. *Sexualities*, *28*(1–2), 450–69; Wood, K., McCarthy, S., Pitt, H., Randle, M. and Thomas, S. L. (2025). Women's experiences and expectations during the menopause transition: a systematic qualitative narrative review. *Health Promotion International*, *40*(1), daaf005.

34 Bulut, H., Hinchliff, S., Ali, P. and Piercy, H. (2025). Women's experiences of intimate and sexual relationships during menopause: a qualitative synthesis. *Journal of Clinical Nursing*, *34*(5), 1543–54.

35 Kohut, T., Dobson, K. A., Balzarini, R. N., Rogge, R. D., Shaw, A. M., McNulty, J. K., ... and Campbell, L. (2021). But what's your partner up to? Associations between relationship quality and pornography use depend on contextual patterns of use within the couple. *Frontiers in Psychology*, *12*, 661347; Abdi, F., Pakzad, R., Alidost, F., Aghapour, E., Mehrnoush, V. and Banaei, M. (2024). Effect of pornography use on sexual satisfaction: a systematic review and meta-analysis. *Journal of Addictive Diseases*, 1–18.

36 Avis, N. E., Colvin, A., Karlamangla, A. S., Crawford, S., Hess, R., Waetjen, L. E., ... and Greendale, G. A. (2017). Change in sexual functioning over the menopausal transition: results from the Study of Women's Health Across the Nation. *Menopause*, *24*(4), 379–90.

37 Avis, N. E., Zhao, X., Johannes, C. B., Ory, M., Brockwell, S. and Greendale, G. A. (2005). Correlates of sexual function among multi-ethnic middle-aged women: results from the Study of Women's Health Across the Nation (SWAN). *Menopause, 12*(4), 385–8.
38 Smith, R. L., Gallicchio, L. and Flaws, J. A. (2017). Factors affecting sexual function in midlife women: results from the midlife Women's Health Study. *Journal of Women's Health, 26*(9), 923–32.
39 Mark, K. P. and Lasslo, J. A. (2018). Maintaining sexual desire in long-term relationships: a systematic review and conceptual model. *The Journal of Sex Research, 55*(4–5), 563–81.
40 Bulut, H., Hinchliff, S., Ali, P. and Piercy, H. (2025). Women's experiences of intimate and sexual relationships during menopause: a qualitative synthesis. *Journal of Clinical Nursing, 34*(5), 1543–54.
41 Wolfman, W., Krakowsky, Y. and Fortier, M. (2021). Guideline No. 422d: menopause and sexuality. *Journal of Obstetrics and Gynaecology Canada, 43*(11), 1334–41.

Acknowledgements

Joe Warner, Summer 2025

Firstly, thank you to my agent, **Oscar Janson-Smith**, for believing in me and this project – and for your unwavering support from our very first meeting. To **Victoria Roddam**, my editorial director at Sheldon Press – thank you for your faith in me, your belief in the mission, and for bringing this book to life. To **Jen Campbell**, our brilliant senior project editor, for her skill and care in guiding us to the finish line. Thank you.

And, of course, to my co-author **Rob Kemp**, who gave me my first taste of consumer magazine craft during work experience at *Men's Health* back in the summer of 2003 – so, in many ways, my entire career is all his fault. Jokes aside, the inspiration for this project came from his brilliant books on fatherhood – *The Expectant Dad's Survival Guide* and *The New Dad's Survival Guide* – which I've gifted to many friends over the years, making some glow with joy, others go as white as a sheet.

This book would not have been possible without the generosity, insight, expertise and personal stories shared by so many remarkable people. I owe them all a debt of gratitude I hope to repay one day. Here they are, in the order in which they appear:

Dr Victoria Felkar, for illuminating the complex, interconnected reality of hormonal health and for bringing clarity, depth and intelligence to one of the most misunderstood aspects of human health. **Kate Rowe-Ham**, for showing that midlife strength starts with honesty and for empowering women to take back control of their bodies, their confidence and their relationships, one rep and realization at a time. **Christine D'Ercole**, for proving that even world champions can be blindsided by the menopause, for speaking out with honesty and strength that no woman should have to face it alone, and for pushing me through countless Peloton Power Zone rides when my body was screaming to stop pedalling.

Dr Jeff Foster, for calling out the confusion and complacency around men's health, and for helping men take their symptoms seriously, reclaim their energy, and change the story before it's too late.

Mike Bates, for his inspirational work in redefining midlife not as a crisis but as a turning point, and for sharing his incredible story with honesty, strength and purpose to help other men find theirs. **Dr Ben Davis**, for cutting through the testosterone hype with straight-talking clarity, and for reminding men that strength, energy and confidence start with healthier habits, not quick-fix hacks.

Nigel Taberner, for translating decades of high-stakes negotiation into powerful, practical tools for everyday relationships, and for showing how compassion and curiosity can defuse even the most emotionally charged moments. **Jaz Ampaw-Farr**, for sharing how real connection begins with presence, patience and a willingness to listen, and for being one of the most inspiring and supportive people I've had the pleasure to interview. You're a force of nature – in the very best way. **Jessica Barac**, for turning her difficult experiences into powerful, practical wisdom, and for showing that with the right words, a little patience and a lot of presence, even the toughest moments can bring people closer.

Rachel Mason, for her extraordinary bravery in sharing what so many women go through in silence, and for channelling her life-changing experience into a one-woman mission to inform, support and empower others. **Dr Philippa Kaye**, for championing personalized, compassionate menopause care, and for reminding us that good medicine starts with listening, understanding and respecting every woman's individual journey. **Caitlin Murray**, for speaking the truth about motherhood, mental health and midlife with guts, humour and honesty, and for reminding us that being believed is one of the greatest acts of love.

Oliver Patrick, for redefining what resilience really means – not just bouncing back, but building better foundations – because managing stress isn't about hacks or heroics, but daily habits that help you stay in control. **Nick Littlehales**, for changing the way we think about sleep, and for proving that proper recovery isn't about chasing eight hours of perfection, but creating simple, sustainable rhythms that actually work in the real world.

Rhiannon Lambert, for bringing warmth, clarity and kindness to the often overwhelming world of nutrition and for showing that eating well doesn't have to mean restriction, rules or stress, but can be simple, joyful and free from guilt. **Nigel Denby**, for his straight-talking approach to midlife eating, and for empowering women to ditch diet myths and take back control with confidence, clarity and common sense. **Professor Emeran Mayer**, for his decades of pioneering work unlocking the secrets of the gut–brain connection, and for showing us that better digestion, stronger immunity and a happier mind all begin in the same place. **Ian Marber**, for his clear and pragmatic take on nutrition and supplements, and for blending evidence and experience with just the right dose of wit, humour and Taylor Swift references.

Dr Alyssa Olenick, for flipping the script on exercise – to make fitness feel like freedom, not punishment – and for helping women let go of guilt, trust their bodies and train in ways that build strength, confidence and self-belief. **Melanie Bauer**, for sharing her extraordinary journey with courage, warmth and wisdom, and for reminding us all that strength, pride and passion can be reclaimed at any age and on your own terms. **Sarah Louise Ryan**, for cutting through the clichés to show what real connection takes, and for helping couples rebuild intimacy through empathy, honesty, and the small everyday acts that keep love alive.

And extra special thanks to **Dr Louise Newson**, for transforming the menopause conversation with relentless drive, for sharing her own perimenopause story, and for so generously giving her time to check copy, offer encouragement, and champion this project from the start. Thank you. Also **Kate Muir**, for fearlessly changing the national conversation on the menopause, and for using truth, tenacity and personal storytelling to empower a generation of women to reclaim their health and happiness. Thank you for backing this project with such enthusiasm and encouragement.

And **Dr Stacy Sims**, for transforming the way the world understands female physiology, and for beating the drum that women are not small men and deserve training, fuelling and support that reflect their biology. Thank you for proving that strength, science and self-belief go hand in hand.

Although I didn't interview them for this book, I'd like to acknowledge conversations with **Dr Carole Hooven**, evolutionary biologist and author of *Testosterone: The Story of the Hormone that Dominates and Divides Us*; **Baz Moffat**, co-author of *The Female Body Bible* and chief executive of The Well HQ; and **Dr Abbie Smith-Ryan**, a leading expert in exercise physiology and sports nutrition. Each conversation played a valuable role in helping shape the early ideas behind this project.

I'd also like to thank **Jon Lipsey**, my longtime collaborator. While not directly involved in this project, it wouldn't have been possible without the help, advice and extraordinary talent he's shared with me over more than 15 years of working together. His decision to hire me as a staff writer at *Men's Fitness* changed my life – giving a bored business journalist his dream job, and opening the door to so many incredible projects, adventures and people.

Finally, to my mum, **Chrissy**, and my dad, **Jonathan** – thank you for your love, patience and support, and for always being there when I needed it most.

To my son, **Jack** – you're far too young for any of this: we've got to cover where babies come from first. But when the time is right, I hope you find this book helpful. Us boys have got to do better, baby – nothing will change until we do.

And to **Lucy**, thank you – for patiently showing me how little I really understood about women's health and the menopause, for sharing podcasts, articles and the stories of so many women who've been misunderstood and mistreated. For reading every page as I wrote it, for your honesty, your advice, and all the ways you've supported and encouraged me – not just through this book, but from the moment we met. It means more to me than you'll ever know.

Joe x

Rob Kemp, July 2025

It wouldn't have been possible without the following supporting cast. Thanks to **Oscar Janson-Smith** for his faith in us and his determination to bring this book to life, and to **Victoria Roddam** at John Murray Press for her support, encouragement and guidance throughout. And a thank you to **Jen Campbell** at Sheldon for her editing, feedback and guidance.

For their advice and contributions, not all of which made the final cut but were massively helpful all the same, I'd like to thank **Dr Nicky Keay**, not only for the insight into the myths around the menopause but for a crash course in Greek mythology in the process. To **Kelly Casperson MD** for telling it like it is and helping millions

Acknowledgements

of women realize that they're not broken. To **Kathy Abernethy, Dr Angela Wright, Deborah Garlick**, founder of Henpicked, and **Lucy Cavendish** for their expertise and for answering even my daftest of questions. **To Diane Danzebrink** at Menopause Support UK for being a pioneer in getting men involved in the menopause conversation.

In my research for this book I have to thank Men's Shed. Also **Ben Towell** and **Matt Balfour** – consultants championing menopause awareness among men. **Nigel Carlos** and **Thomas Elle** at Men's Circle for putting the menopause on the agenda in the workplace and among men's support groups. And to **Katherine Selby** along with **David Threlfall-Sykes, Raj Bains** and **Zoe Shackleton** (all at Huddersfield Town FC) for allowing me to see how forward-thinking firms are raising awareness about the menopause and its implications for employees and employers.

For their candid conversations about their menopause experiences I must thank **Kevin, Bryan, Jane, John Collins, Carol Collins, James Culver, Steve Mato, Nicola Goodship-Leonard** and, of course, my wife, **Amanda**, who said from the get-go that this was a much-needed book – I'm just sorry we never got to use your title suggestion of 'Angry Birds'.

Most of all I want to thank my co-author, colleague, supporter and friend **Joe Warner** whose work – not least of all on my copy – has been incredible. Your amazing idea has come to fruition, Joe – it's been a privilege to be a part of the journey.

Rob

Index

4-7-8 breathing, 157

active listening, 85–88
acupuncture, 134
adrenaline, 75, 153
age of menopause onset, 6
alcohol, 167, 183–184
alternative therapies, 134–135
American English terminology, xiv
anger
  controlling your own, 75–78
  responding to, 73–75
antidepressants, 100, 105–106, 132–133
anxiety, 7–8, 24
aromatherapy, 155
ashwagandha, 187

behaviour changes, responding suitably, 40–42
belly fat, 203, 211
bench for exercise, 209
bent-over row exercise, 206–207
beta blockers, 133
blood tests, 99, 135–136
body confidence, 142–146
body-identical hormones, 119
body language, 88
body mass index (BMI), 145
bones, 203
box breathing, 76, 157
brain fog, 23–24, 36, 204
breast cancer, 123–125
breathing exercises, 76, 156–157
brush-off bingo, 104–105

caffeine, 167
calcium, 187
calming strategies, 76–78, 156–160, 169
carbohydrates, 173

cardiovascular exercise, 211–212
  see also exercise
chemotherapy, 111
clonidine, 134
clothing for exercise, 200–201
cognitive behavioural therapy (CBT), 134, 155, 165
coil (contraceptive), 133
communication
  diffusing arguments, 80–81
  responding to angry comments, 73–75
  saying the right things, 83–88, 92–93
  saying the wrong things, 88–89
  about sex, 231–233
  suitable time and place for, 82–83
  tactics, 90–91
  tone and body language, 88
  traffic light list, 93–94
complementary therapies, 134–135
compounded bioidentical hormones, 119
contraceptive coil, 133
contraceptive pill, 125, 133
cortisol, 13, 24, 49, 75, 153, 187
creatine, 187–189
curcumin, 189

deadlifts, 205
diagnosis of menopause, 135–136
dietary supplements, 186–191
diets *see also* food
  faddy, 176
  healthy, 175, 176–180
  Mediterranean diet, 176–177, 178–179
digestive system, 184–185
divorce, 8, 32, 34–35

doctors
  appointments with, 102–105
  dismissiveness, 104–105
  limitations, 98–101, 130
  second opinions, 106
  when to see, 96, 101–102
dumbbells, 209

early menopause (ages 40–45), 17–18, 97
early signs of menopause, 5, 35–36
education about menopause, 6
erectile dysfunction, 223
exercise, 155, 194–196, 214–215
  clothing for, 200–201
  and eating, 199–200
  equipment, 209
  high-intensity interval training (HIIT), 197, 199, 210–212
  low-intensity steady-state (LISS) cardio, 197, 212–213
  myths, 196
  overcoming excuses, 218–220
  plyometric training, 197, 214
  Priority Pyramid, 197–198
  strength training, 196–197, 198–199, 202–210
  training programme, 216–218
exercise mats, 210

fasted training, 199–200
fats in food, 173–174, 178
fermented foods, 185–186
fertility, effect of TRT, 61–62
fibre, 178, 185
follicle-stimulating hormone (FSH), 13
food
  avoiding weight gain, 180–182
  cravings, 182–183
  effect on gut microbiome, 185–186
  and exercise, 199–200
  faddy diets, 176
  healthy diets, 175, 176–180
  Mediterranean diet, 176–177, 178–179
  nutrients, 172–175, 177–178
four pillars of health, 146

gabapentin, 134
GPs
  appointments with, 102–105
  dismissiveness, 104–105
  limitations, 98–101, 130
  second opinions, 106
  when to see, 96, 101–102
gut microbiome, 184–185

health, 159–160, 175, 176–180
healthcare systems, 96
  limitations, 98–101, 130
  online, 109–110
heart health, 211
herbal remedies, 135
high-intensity interval training (HIIT), 197, 199, 210–212
home gym, 209
hormones, 12–27, 31–32, 117–118 *see also* HRT (hormone replacement therapy)
  involved in anger, 75
  lifecycle, 15
  manufactured, 119
  in men, 48–50, 52, 57–64
  and sleep, 165
  stress, 13, 24, 49, 75, 152–153
hormone-suppressing therapies, 111
hot flushes, 23, 35–36, 167
HRT (hormone replacement therapy), 116–117
  advantages, 121–123
  age to start at, 121
  alternatives to, 132–135
  association with breast cancer, 123–125
  deciding against, 131–136
  delivery methods, 118–119
  fine-tuning, 129–130
  myths, 125–126, 130

risks, 123–125
side effects, 128–129
timing of effects, 120
for weight issues, 145–146
hypoactive sexual desire disorder (HSDD), 121

individual differences, 99
induced menopause, 110–112
insulin, 13, 49
insurance, 107
intimacy issues, 8–9
IUDs (intrauterine devices), 133

journalling, 157

kettlebells, 210

libido
  increased, 42–43
  loss of, 25, 37, 121, 226–230
  loss of in men, 51
listening skills, 85–88
low-intensity steady-state (LISS) cardio, 197, 212–213
luteinizing hormone (LH), 13

magnesium, 190
'manopause', 49–50
marriage breakdowns, 8–9, 32, 34–35
masturbation, 227
medical gaslighting, 101
medical insurance, 107
medical menopause, 110–112
medical support *see also* private treatment
  advocating for, 99, 103–104
  appointments, 102–105
  online healthcare, 109–110
  second opinions, 106
  signs that she needs, 96, 101–102
meditation, 157
Mediterranean diet, 176–177, 178–179

melatonin, 13, 25
men, changes during midlife, 43–44, 45–64
menopause specialists, 107–108
  online, 109–110
menopause stage, definition, 4
menstruation, irregular periods, 37–38
micro recovery moments (MRMs), 169
microbiome, 184–185
midlife, changes in men, 43–44, 45–64
midlife crisis, 52–55
Midlife MOT, 147–148
mindfulness, 157–158
minerals, 186–190
Mirena, 133
misdiagnoses, 100
misinformation, 10
mood swings, 36
Mounjaro, 127–128
muscles, 174, 187–189, 203 *see also* strength training

napping, 168
negotiation, 83–84, 92–93
nerve endings, 36–37
night sweats, 23, 35–36, 167
norepinephrine, 153

oestrogen, 12–14, 18–20, 117–118
omega-3 fatty acids, 190–191
online healthcare, 109–110
ovaries, removal, 110–111
overwhelm, 162
Ozempic, 127–128

panic attacks, 24
perimenopause stage, 4, 16
periods, irregular, 37–38
personality changes, 38
physical activity, 155, 194–196, 214–215
  clothing for, 200–201
  and eating, 199–200

equipment, 209
high-intensity interval training (HIIT), 197, 199, 210–212
low-intensity steady-state (LISS) cardio, 197, 212–213
myths, 196
overcoming excuses, 218–220
plyometric training, 197, 214
Priority Pyramid, 197–198
strength training, 196–197, 198–199, 202–210
training programme, 216–218
plyometric training, 197, 214
postmenopause stage, 4, 16
premature menopause (before 40), 18
premenopause stage, hormone levels, 15–16
private treatment, 106–107
for TRT, 58, 60, 62, 63–64
progesterone, 12–13, 14, 118–119
progressive muscle relaxation (PMR), 158
protein, 173, 174, 177, 190
and exercise, 200
psychological symptoms of menopause, 20–21, 23–24

questions to ask, 84–85
of the GP, 103

radiation therapy, 111
relaxation, 76–78, 156–160, 169
resistance bands, 209
responding to angry comments, 73–75
responding to behavioural changes, 40–42
rhodiola rosea, 191
routine, 82, 159–160, 169
exercise programme, 216–218
mealtime, 181

scent, changes in, 38
schools, teaching about menopause, 6

second mountain, 53–54, 55–56
second opinions, 106
sex, 222
dysfunction, 121, 223–226
improving, 230–233
increased interest in, 42–43
intimacy issues, 8–9
loss of interest for men, 51
loss of interest in, 25, 37, 121, 226–230
shoulder press, 206
skin, different scent, 38
skin sensations, 36–37
sleep, 24–25, 158, 162–169
sports bras, 201
squats, 204–205
strength training, 196–197, 198–199, 202–210
stress, 149–158, 186, 187
suicidal thoughts, 32
supplements, 186–191
surgical menopause, 18, 110–112
symptoms of menopause, 20–25, 33–34
early signs, 5, 35–36
gathering evidence, 102
needing medical support, 96, 101–102
synthetic hormones, 119

testosterone, 13, 14, 25, 118
in men, 48–50, 52, 57–64
testing, 57–59
therapy, 59–64, 121
tone of voice, 88
traffic light list, 93–94
training programme, 216–218
TRT (testosterone replacement treatment), 59–64

ultra-processed foods (UPFs), 186
Unify charity, 47

vagina, soreness, 37
vaginal dryness, 25, 223

vaginal hormones, 120, 226
vasomotor symptoms, 23, 35–36
Viagra, 125
virtuous cycle, 146–147
vitamin D, 189

waist-to-height ratio, 145
Wegovy, 127–128

weight gain, 142–146, 180–182
weightlifting, 196–197, 198–199, 202–210
weight loss, 213
weight-loss drugs, 127–128

yoga, 134–135